CASE STUDIES in LAW and NURSING

CASE STUDIES
in LAW and NURSING

A course book for Project 2000 training

ANN P. YOUNG

Deputy Registrar, Nightingale and Guy's College of Health

CHAPMAN & HALL
London · Glasgow · New York · Tokyo · Melbourne · Madras

Published by Chapman & Hall, 2-6 Boundary Row, London SE1 8HN

Chapman & Hall, 2-6 Boundary Row, London SE1 8HN, UK

Blackie Academic & Professional, Wester Cleddens Road, Bishopbriggs, Glasgow G64 2NZ, UK

Chapman & Hall, 29 West 35th Street, New York NY10001, USA

Chapman & Hall Japan, Thomson Publishing Japan, Hirakawacho Nemoto Building, 6F, 1-7-11 Hirakawa-cho, Chiyoda-ku, Tokyo 102, Japan

Chapman & Hall Australia, Thomas Nelson Australia, 102 Dodds Street, South Melbourne, Victoria 3205, Australia

Chapman & Hall India, R. Seshadri, 32 Second Main Road, CIT East, Madras 600 035, India

Distributed in the USA and Canada by Singular Publishing Group Inc., 4284 41st Street, San Diego, California 92105

First edition 1992

Typeset in 10/12pt Garamond ITC by Best-set Typesetter Ltd., Hong Kong

Printed in Great Britain by Richard Clays Ltd, Bungay

ISBN 0 412 44130 6   1 56593 034 7 (USA)

A catalogue record for this book is available from the British Library

Contents

Acknowledgements

Permission to reproduce material is gratefully acknowledged from HMSO, the United Kingdom Central Council, Blackwell, Oxford University Press, McDonald and Evans Ltd, Penguin Books, Prentice Hall, Professional and Scientific Publications and Macmillan Magazines Ltd.

My thanks go to Sarah Mobbs and Cally Ward for their specialist advice, to my students at Guy's Hospital for trying out and commenting on the material in this book, to Linda Pullen for typing the manuscript, to John Tingle for his legal expertise and to my husband Robert for his continuing enthusiasm and help.

Preface

Case Studies in Law and Nursing is not a conventional book, more a learning pack. There are now several textbooks in existence which give detailed material on law and nursing for reference purposes and provide for the nurse at any stage of her career. The problems for the nurse in training is to sort out what legal knowledge is essential to her practice as its sheer volume can be overwhelming. The situation has been further complicated by a change in the Nurses Rules (1989) so that 'an understanding of the requirements of legislation relevant to the practice of nursing' is now a necessary outcome for registration of those undertaking Project 2000 training. Of course, those preparing students for registration under previous training schemes will have included a certain amount of relevant legal material, but this topic must now be more clearly and obviously addressed by both students and teachers – and be applied to a rather different range of circumstances.

The Nurses Rules (1983) saw achievement of the competencies required for registration as a shared responsibility between student and training institution, and this philosophy is continued and extended in the Project 2000 course guidelines. The textbook does not normally promote active participation of the reader. That conventionally has to be achieved through tutorial classes or the setting of written work which then requires marking! In either case, a teacher with legal and nursing knowledge is required and unfortunately such experts are rather few and far between.

Case Studies in Law and Nursing aims to resolve these difficulties. The patient or client is central to the book's approach with legal information being incorporated to illustrate various aspects of care. Students can work through the book either alone or in groups as active participation is required both in attempting to answer questions pertinent to each case study and in undertaking various activities that will help to reinforce what has been learnt and enable the student to see how the law is interpreted in reality. While the book can stand alone in that the questions posed are answered and discussed in the text, the student should be encouraged to refer to other sources as well and a comprehensive list of recommended reading is included for this purpose.

The book has been planned around the framework of Project 2000. Situations involving both community and institutional care are presented throughout as well as covering the four branches of nursing: adult, mental, mental handicap and children. Part One, the Common Foundation Programme, should be completed before proceeding further as a wide range of legal material is presented to the student at a basic level. This will then be extended in Parts Two and Three in addition to the inclusion of some new material. The chapters in Part One can be tackled in any order and work on them can be continued even after the student has entered her Branch Programme.

There is a specific chapter for each Branch. However, the law may be seen as a unifying component of Project 2000 training and could well be one area where shared learning between the Branches can take place. Students may therefore benefit by studying the other case studies and identifying the common legal principles that are included.

Part Three, Preparation for Registration, should again be completed by all students. The material presented requires a more analytical approach and a greater depth of legal knowledge, thus encouraging a progression of skill in handling legal concepts throughout the course of the book.

The overall aim is to make learning about the law fun. Students undertaking other courses of training and staff whose training included minimal legal input may also enjoy this book. As a teacher myself, I certainly hope that tutors will find it a useful way to tackle this aspect of nurse training.

Ann P. Young

Note: For simplicity, in most cases, the nurse is referred to in the female gender.

How to use this book

Working on your own

Case Studies in Law and Nursing can be used as a distance learning pack. Even used on its own, the book will provide you with a very workable knowledge of the law that you can apply to nursing. Whichever Branch you are following (or area in which you are working for those not on a Project 2000 course) it is recommended that you look at all the case studies. It is surprising how aspects of the law relating to one situation can be relevant to another, and, as a learning exercise it is useful to explore this. For additional suggestions, see Instructions to Teachers. You will also find that you gain more from this book if you use a reference book alongside it, e.g. Young, A.P. (1989) *Legal Problems in Nursing Practice*, 2nd edition, Harper and Row.

Working with other students

Whether you prefer working on your own or with others is a very individual thing. On your own, you can go at your own pace and have total freedom of choice as to the order in which you do the case studies (within the constraints laid down below). However, there are a number of advantages to working with others. Two or more minds often make the going easier by sharing knowledge and experience in both nursing and life. You may decide to tackle the questions together or to attempt them on your own and then come together to discuss your answers. A joint discussion of the answers in the book in the light of your attempts and other reading of textbooks, journals and newspapers will often reinforce learning and clarify points of difficulty.

Undertaking the activities can also be rewarding. Where visits are involved it can be easier to do these with a partner if you are not feeling very confident or students can choose to visit a number of locations with a subsequent comparing of notes of differences encountered.

Choosing the order of work

It is advisable that each part of the book is completed before proceeding further. This is because the level of difficulty increases throughout the book, as well as later parts relying on the acquisition of knowledge from earlier case studies. However, within each part you can choose the order in which you work. For example, you may wish to pick a topic from Part One that particularly interests you in order to get underway. In Part Two, you could tackle the chapter relating to your own Branch before exploring how the law can be applied in other specialities.

Using resource material

This falls into two categories, the case study answers and external material.

For each case study the answers are found at the end, grouped together rather than after each question in the main body of the chapter. Although this means flicking the pages from questions to answers, students who have tried out this format state that if the answer is immediately under the question, it is too tempting to read straight on without even trying to answer what is asked! So try to answer each question posed. You can do this purely from your own knowledge and experience or you can use other sources such as textbooks.

Using the first approach, you may well find that initially all you can do is hazard a guess, perhaps using a common-sense approach. To compare your answer with the legal ones can be illuminating as the law does not always appear to be either logical or sensible! However, as you proceed in the book you will find that you are able to build on previous learning. At this point the value of the book's answers may well be their inclusion of rationale and some of the 'ifs' and 'buts' always found in the law.

If you wish to look for the answers in other textbooks, there is a list of useful references at the end of each chapter. This is certainly a very active way of learning factual material but do remember to also learn the skills of being critical of the law and how it is implemented, particularly in Parts Two and Three.

Undertaking the activities

The case studies could be completed without undertaking the activities. While it is accepted that time may be limited, it is strongly recommended that the activities are not omitted. The whole purpose of including law in a nursing programme is so that the nurse can apply her knowledge and understand the relevance of decisions that have legal significance within a work setting. She can only do this by integrating theory and practice.

As suggested above, working with other students rather than on your own can make the activities easier and more enjoyable. The activities could also be distributed amongst a group of students although subsequent sharing cannot totally replace first hand experience.

Do not forget certain ground rules when visiting departments or asking for information. Always explain who you are and why you are there. If you have arrived at an inconvenient moment, withdraw and return later or go elsewhere. Be sensitive to other people's needs and problems. Maintain confidentiality. Staff are usually very interested in what students are doing and put themselves out to be helpful. You may get a lot more out of the activities than you anticipate!

INSTRUCTIONS TO TEACHERS

Preparing the students

Both initiating and maintaining interest in the law as applied to nursing are problematic as to timing and technique.

From personal experience, it is better not to start the input on law right at the beginning of the course as the student lacks any relevant conceptual frameworks. However it does link with a number of other subject areas, most obviously ethics and professional studies, so could be initiated in conjunction with these.

The techniques that prove most effective are the topic of this book. The introductory quiz triggers great interest and enthusiasm. I know! I have used it with very disparate groups with students working either singly or in groups. An additional means of arousing interest could be for the students to undertake a legal/health media watch.

Before commencing the case studies, it is advisable to discuss with the students in detail what you expect from them with regard to both the questions and activities, for example in relation to feedback and sharing of experiences. Consideration must be given to stating clear time allowances for the completion of work.

Teaching approaches

A number of approaches can be used, even by the teacher who does not feel very confident in the legal arena.

Seminars will probably be the cornerstone for the legal component of the course. Student-initiated discussion of the case studies will help to reinforce learning that has already occurred (see Instructions to Students). As the course proceeds, sharing between students undertaking different Branch programmes will become increasingly important. Discussion of the Part Three case studies should assist with the integration of the legal programme with other parts of the course.

Tutorials will be needed at intervals to provide unification of the main legal topics. A list of these with reference to the relevant questions and answers in the case studies is given in Appendix C. In addition teachers are recommended to use my two other books *Legal Problems in Nursing Practice* (1989) and *Law and Professional Conduct in Nursing* (1991).

Your educational establishment will probably have a surprising number of staff resources, not necessarily experts in law but in their own specialist areas of nursing. Team teaching may be the best way of tapping this resource. For example, looking at the topic of consent, teachers in psychiatric, paediatric and accident and emergency nursing will all have useful perspectives.

Outside speakers will add interest to the course. Your health authority will be able to provide some expertise, for example in data protection, health and safety at work, union organization, the Mental Health Act and personnel and employment policies. Police, social workers and legal personnel may also contribute. Be aware that these people, while being experts in their areas, will not necessarily have the skills to apply their knowledge to nursing and should therefore be used in addition to, not instead of, the other teaching approaches.

Assessment of learning

As a knowledge of the law relevant to nursing is one of the outcomes required under Rule 18A, assessment of this knowledge seems appropriate. My view is that such assessment should use a variety of tools, both conventional and imaginative.

The Foundation Programme could be assessed by the use of diaries of clinical experience and visits with the student having to identify the legal significance of what she observes. During Branch Programmes seminar presentations of critical incidents with legal relevance can be used to assess the student's ability in analysis.

Towards the end of the course, an extended essay on a particular aspect of the law might demonstrate a critical appraisal of how the law is applied to nursing situations.

Introduction

The following quiz forms the major part of the introduction. There is a glossary of legal terms included to check words used in the quiz of whose precise meaning you are not sure. (You can also refer back to the glossary as you work through the book.)

WHAT DO YOU KNOW ABOUT THE LAW?

1. If you see a crime being committed, do you have to report it?
2. If the police ask you to accompany them to the police station, do you have to go?
3. If you buy goods that turn out to be faulty, what legislation protects your rights?
4. What is the difference between a magistrate and a justice of the peace (JP)?
5. If you want to be represented in court, do you approach a solicitor or a barrister?
6. What is wrong with the statement, 'Trespassers will be prosecuted'?
7. If you are physically threatened by an individual, how much force can you use to deter him?
8. You leave a pile of bricks on the public footpath outside your house for a week and a pedestrian falls over them. Does he have a claim against you?
9. What is an employment contract?
10. What is the highest court in the United Kingdom?
11. What is negligence?
12. If you think your doctor has been negligent in treating you, what is the time limit within which you must start suing him for the injuries you have sustained?
13. On visiting a friend in hospital, you fall and twist your ankle as a result of slipping on a wet floor that has just been washed. Do you have a claim against the hospital?
14. Is an employer responsible for the wrong-doings of his employees?
15. Anyone over 18 years old can make a will. What other characteristic must he possess?

16. What is an injunction?
17. Is it illegal to attempt to commit suicide?
18. What is the responsibility of the ombudsman (health service commissioner)?
19. A colleague tells your workmakes that you have AIDS. Can you sue him for slander?
20. Is it illegal for a doctor to divulge confidential information to another person about your medical condition?
21. If you carry a donor card, does this automatically mean that your organs (assuming they are healthy) can be used after your death?
22. In what circumstances does a death have to be reported to a coroner?
23. Can a child consent to medical treatment?
24. What is a Controlled Drug?
25. When does a nurse have a legal right to refuse to look after a patient?

ANSWERS

1. No.
2. No, unless they arrest you.
3. Sale of Goods Act 1979, Trade Description Act 1968.
4. None.
5. A solicitor.
6. Only crimes can lead to prosecution and trespass is a civil wrong, not a crime.
7. Such force as is reasonably proportionate to that being used against you.
8. Yes, probably, unless you had warned the pedestrian.
9. A legally binding agreement between employer and employee involving offer and acceptance.
10. The House of Lords.
11. Failure to take reasonable care to avoid acts or omissions that cause harm to your 'neighbour'.
12. Three years from the time of the negligent act or when the effects of the injury become apparent.
13. No, if reasonable steps were taken to warn you of the danger. Otherwise, yes.
14. Yes, if someone was harmed during the carrying out of the employee's normal duties (by vicarious liability). No, if outside this remit or a criminal activity.
15. A sound mind.
16. A court order forbidding or ordering the carrying out of some act.
17. No.
18. To investigate complaints by members of the public relating to health care.
19. Unlikely if it is true or if it is not made public.
20. No.
21. No. Those either owning or in possession of your body have the legal right to decide.

22. Any death that is unexplained, in suspicious circumstances, during operation or shortly after admission to hospital.
23. Yes, in an emergency if he has sufficient understanding.
24. A drug so named under the Misuse of Drugs Act, for example morphine, diamorphine (heroin), pethidine.
25. If she has a conscientious objection under the Abortion Act or if it would involve participation in a crime or a negligent act.

SCORING

Questions 1–8 reflected general knowledge.
Questions 9–16 some legal knowledge required.
Questions 17–25 some medical/nursing knowledge also necessary.

If you did not get many right, do not be disheartened. Read on!

Glossary of legal terms

Action:	civil proceedings in a court of law.
Actus reus:	the guilty act.
Assault:	threat of violence against the person.
Barrister:	legally trained person who acts for the defendant or plaintif.
Battery:	carrying out of violence against the person.
Bill:	draft act presented to Parliament.
Case law:	judge made law created by referring to previous similar cases.
Children:	persons under 14 years in England and Wales.
Civil wrong:	a wrong perpetrated by one individual on another.
Common law:	non statute law.
Consent:	legal defence for trespass.
Contract:	legal agreement.
Coroner:	a legal or medical practitioner with authority to enquire into sudden, unexpected or suspicious death.
Crime:	offence committed against the public, punishable by the State Crown Prosecution Service: a body headed by the Director of Public Prosecutions for screening which serious legal cases are taken to court.
Damages:	an award of compensation.
Defamation:	making public untrue and derogatory statements about an individual.
Defendant:	the accused, the person who is sued or prosecuted.
Delict:	Scottish term for tort.

European Court of Human Rights:	supreme court in Europe dealing with those matters that are separate from an individual's own country.
Expert witness:	an expert who can give his opinion on a subject in court.
Green paper:	consultative document on suggested legislation.
Holograph:	a will in a person's own handwriting with no witnesses, legal in Scotland.
Illegal:	breaking the criminal law.
Injunction:	a court order requiring someone to do or refrain from doing something.
Judge:	experienced legal person hearing cases in the higher courts.
Juveniles:	persons under 17 years in England and Wales.
Libel:	defamation in written form.
Magistrate:	Justice of the Peace, a lay person hearing cases in a magistrates court.
Mens rea:	the criminal intention.
Minor:	a person under 18 years.
Negligence:	causing harm to a person to whom a duty is owed either by doing some act which a reasonable person would not do or not doing what a reasonable person would have done.
Plaintiff:	the person who brings a civil action for suffering harm.
Pupil:	in Scotland, a boy under 14 years, a girl under 12 years.
Sheriff:	legal person hearing certain criminal and civil cases in Scotland.
Slander:	defamation in spoken form; in Scotland a verbal injury comparable to battery.
Solicitor:	a legally trained person who acts for the individual outside of the court system (except magistrates court).
Statute:	act of Parliament.
Statutory instruments, rules or orders:	system of delegated legislation.
Subpoena:	a legal order to attend court.

Tort: a civil wrong.

Trespass: invasion of personal territory.

Tribunal: a forum for legally settling disputes between the individual and the appropriate authority.

Unlawful: breaching civil law.

Vicarious liability: legal responsibility of the employer for its employees' torts.

White paper: document containing detailed proposals of suggested legislation.

PART ONE

Common Foundation

Programme – Level 1

Respecting the individual 1

Mrs Rose Bolton is an elderly lady of 84 years. She was widowed two years ago when her husband died suddenly after a stroke. Her daughter and son-in-law give her some support but live ten miles away and have their own teenage family to care for. However they visit approximately monthly and do some cleaning and maintenance jobs for her. Rose has some disability and pain due to arthritis and also gets breathless on exertion. She refuses any help apart from that offered by her family. However she will occasionally let the district nurse into the house and accept assistance with a bath and hairwash. On other visits the nurse is told to go away without Rose even opening the door.

Can the nurse insist on being allowed entry?

Question 1.1

Activity 1.1
Find out who is legally entitled to enter a person's home and in what circumstances.

One Monday morning, Rose's daughter phones the nurse to express great anxiety about her mother. On arriving at the house, the nurse is relieved that on this occasion Rose opens the door to her, but she is shocked by the condition in which she finds her. She looks unkempt and smells strongly of urine. Although coherent, she speaks in abusive terms about her daughter, accusing her of being interfering and bossy. It also takes her some time to get her breath back after letting the nurse enter. After some discussion Rose admits that she is not feeling very well and agrees to the nurse contacting the general practitioner.

Case Studies in Law and Nursing,
Ann P. Young.
Published in 1992 by
Chapman & Hall, London
ISBN 0 412 44130 6.

Question 1.2 If Rose had stated that she did not want the doctor contacted, would the nurse have had to abide by this?

Activity 1.2
Read the UKCC's leaflet on *Confidentiality*, pp. 3–7.

On seeing Mrs Bolton the doctor is also concerned as to her general health. He contacts the daughter and son-in-law to inform them of this and strongly advises that Rose be admitted to hospital for care and assessment.

Question 1.3 Is the doctor breaching confidentiality by discussing Rose's situation with the relatives rather than with his patient?
Can a patient prevent this happening?

However, when this is suggested to Rose, she is adamant that she will not go into hospital. She states that if she is going to die, she would rather die at home. The daughter fears that for her mother to stay at home would put an intolerable burden on the whole family as they would feel bound to offer more help. The discussion continues into the next day during which time the doctor liaises with the local geriatric unit for a bed. Once this is available, Rose's daughter and son-in-law collect some of her belongings together, arrange her transport and Rose, still protesting though less forcibly, is taken to hospital.

Have the family and the doctor acted illegally in arranging Rose's admission?

Question 1.4

What part could the nurse have played in this situation to safeguard her patient's interests?

Question 1.5

On arrival in Primrose Ward, a nurse who introduces herself as Fiona welcomes Rose and shows her to her bed area. Fiona suggests to Rose's daughter that she might help her mother to settle in but the daughter says she has to get home and quickly says good-bye to her mother. Fiona helps Rose to unpack making a list of the belongings that she has with her.

Question 1.6   Which items must be listed? What extra precautions must be taken with jewellery and other valuables?

Activity 1.3
Is there a policy on care of patients' property in your health authority? If so, find a copy and read it. If there is no policy, find what paper work has to be completed in relation to a patient's property and valuables.

Fiona then fetches the documentation that has to be completed on a patient's admission. Much of this involves an assessment of the patient's physical, mental and social condition and therefore includes some very personal information. With Rose's contribution and Fiona's observations, a large proportion of this initial nursing assessment is carried out.

Activity 1.4
Find out where the nursing and medical records are kept in a ward of your health authority. What precautions are taken to control access to these in order to maintain confidentiality?

On Primrose Ward, some of the information collected during the nursing assessment has to be put onto a computer to assist with working out what staffing levels are required.

Question 1.7   What material is covered by the Data Protection Act 1984?
What care must Fiona take when transposing confidential information about Rose onto the computer terminal in order to be acting within the law?

For the rest of the day, Rose for the most part sits quietly by her bed and seems rather withdrawn. However, when Fiona and the other nurses come on duty the following morning Rose is wandering around the ward aimlessly, seems not to know where she is and calls Fiona 'Lily' (her daughter's name). She will only sit down when she becomes too breathless to continue walking. As the morning progresses it is noted that she frequently goes to the ward entrance and is only deterred from leaving the ward by the nurses distracting her attention onto something else. After Rose's fifth attempt to leave the ward, the nurses sit her down in a part of the ward that is reasonably visible and put a table in front of her chair in an attempt to stop her getting up. Rose quickly becomes distressed by this and repeatedly shouts 'Let me out! Let me out!' However the nurses have other patients to care for and ignore her cries.

Are the nurses acting legally in preventing Rose from leaving the ward?

Question 1.8

Question 1.9   Are the nurses acting legally in restraining Rose in the way described?

Activity 1.5

Look up a definition of restraint and list some different ways that a patient may be restrained.

At 2 pm after the late shift have received report from the early shift, it is noticed that Rose's chair is empty and on initiating a search, Rose is nowhere to be found in the ward area nor in the immediate environment. Fiona is particularly upset as she feels she should have cared for Rose better and her offer to continue looking for Rose while security is informed is accepted. She decides to look outside the hospital gates and sees Rose on the pavement some way away. As she calls out to her, Rose steps into the road. A car swerves to avoid her and crashes into a lorry travelling in the opposite direction. Rose is unhurt but shaken and on recognizing a familiar face, seems relieved to see Fiona. After asking a nearby shopkeeper to give her name and ward to the police when they arrive, Fiona takes Rose back to the ward.

Question 1.10   Must a witness to an accident or crime give her name and address to the police?

Thirty minutes later two police officers arrive on Primrose Ward and ask to interview Fiona and the sister in charge about the sequence of events leading to the accident.

Do Fiona and the sister have to make statements to the police? What principles should they bear in mind as they make their statements?

Activity 1.6

Study the Sister's statement (below) and identify any faults in it.

'I, Ruth Cole of 10, Barrowgreen Road, am the sister in charge of Primrose Ward, ____ Hospital, and came on duty at 1 pm on May 21st 19 . . . I was told by the morning staff that Mrs Rose Bolton had been admitted the day before with a diagnosis of mild heart failure, urinary infection and arthritis. She had been confused, noisy and uncooperative during the morning and the nurses had kept her in the ward by placing a table in front of her chair. While I was receiving report in the office from the morning staff, Mrs Bolton pushed the table away from her and left the ward. This was discovered as soon as we had finished report. I informed security.'

In the meantime, another nurse, Judith, is allocated to care for Rose who is still confused and restless, but by now extremely breathless and quite cyanosed.

Judith takes a set of baseline observations and finds that Rose's pulse is very fast and irregular. As a matter of urgency she calls the doctor who arrives on the ward 15 minutes later. He prescribes several drugs to be given intravenously and he draws them up in preparation for their administration. When Judith takes Rose's arm, Rose pulls away but by now she is unable to understand what is happening to her in spite of the nurse explaining.

Question 1.12   Are the doctor and nurse legally justified in giving Rose the drugs in spite of not receiving her agreement?

Rose's response to treatment is good and by the following day she is no longer confused. The nurses amend her care plan in view of the medication she has now been prescribed. Judith spends a considerable amount of time explaining to Rose what is being done for her and why, and discussing how the nurses want to help her with her breathing and urinary problems in particular. Rose seems to understand what Judith is suggesting and agrees to cooperate.

Question 1.13   Is it legally necessary for the nurses to involve a patient in formulating his/her care plan?

Activity 1.7

Look at the format used for the care plans in your place of work. Do they have the potential for involving the patient? Is the patient allowed access to his/her care plan?

A week later Rose's two main problems have been resolved although she is still troubled to some extent with arthritic pain and tires easily. She is beginning to grumble about the ward, a sure sign that she is feeling better. She tells the nurses that she wants to go home.

Who decides when a patient is to leave hospital?

Question 1.14

Judith and Fiona both feel that with some support Rose could manage quite well at home and discuss this with the doctor. Rose's daughter is still unhappy about the burden on her family and the professionals accept the need to arrange other support. Surprisingly Rose agrees to accept help from outside the family with the proviso that people do not try to organize her. Home help and district nurse support are suggested.

What legislation enables the provision of home help and district nurse services?

Question 1.15

Activity 1.8
Find out how home help and district nurse services are arranged for a patient being discharged from a hospital in your health authority.

Two weeks after her unwilling admission to hospital, Rose is to be discharged.

Question 1.16   What precautions should the nurses take regarding Rose's property?

Rose returns home, healthier and stronger than she has been for some time. Perhaps the professionals do know best!

Question 1.17   Do you agree?

ANSWERS

Question 1.1

The nurse has no right of entry into a person's home. If she either enters a patient's home without his/her permission or refuses to leave if requested to do so, she becomes a trespasser and can be sued by the occupier. Even if she suspected that Rose was seriously ill and therefore unable to open the door to her, it would be illegal to force an entry. She would have to call the police and leave the decision to them.

Question 1.2

This question poses a recurring problem for the nurse of whether to share with other people personal or private information imparted by a patient.

In Rose's situation where the sharing of information involves another professional caring for the patient there is often an assumption that such breach of confidentiality is legitimate, the other professional, in this case the doctor, being bound by a similar code of professional conduct on this matter as the nurse. However, sharing of information about a patient to someone not entitled to it could lead to a nurse being severely reprimanded by her employer, particularly if she had signed as part of her employment contract that she agreed to maintain confidentiality during the course of her work. Otherwise the legal control over confidential information from a patient is minimal.

The nurse might also reason that *not* to tell the doctor about Rose's deterioration could result in Rose coming to severe harm or dying. The nurse might then be negligent in failing to give proper care to Rose. The patient or her relatives could sue for damages.

Whenever a nurse decides it is in the patient's interests to disclose personal information to another, it seems only right that she should tell the patient of her decision although not legally bound to do so.

Question 1.3

The doctor–patient relationship is bound by a professional code of confidentiality. Therefore on moral grounds it seems to be in breach of this code for the doctor to discuss his patient's condition with other members of the family without the patient's consent. However, as already pointed out, the law lays no requirements on the doctor in this matter. In fact it seems to be assumed that the patient agrees to the doctor acting in this way unless he specifically states that this is not to happen.

Therefore in answer to the second part of the question, the patient could possibly stop the relatives being informed by stating clearly to the doctor that she does not want anyone else given information about her medical condition. However, most patients would be unaware of the necessity of making such a statement. A rather extreme way of preventing a breach of confidence would be to request a court injunction prohibiting such action, but this is rarely practical requiring an awarness of the law, time and money to bring into effect.

Question 1.4

There are only a few instances where a patient can be admitted to hospital against his will.

Under the Mental Health Act 1983 a patient can be admitted for assessment, assessment followed by treatment or for treatment if suffering from a mental disorder of such a nature or degree that this detention is necessary. Rose does not appear to be suffering from a mental disorder, so compulsory admission under this legislation is not appropriate.

The National Assistance Act 1948 contains a section whereby a person can be removed to a place of safety if he is suffering from grave chronic disease or is old and physically incapacitated, is living in insanitary conditions and has no one to care for him nor is able to look after himself. For emergency applications of this nature, the National Assistance (Amendment) Act 1951 would apply. However, a court order is required from a magistrate or sheriff in order for such a removal to be effected. This was not done in Rose's case. A similar order may be required for a person suffering from or carrying certain infectious diseases, again not applicable to Rose.

Question 1.5

The profession frequently discusses the importance of the nurse acting as the patient's advocate, but in reality this is a difficult role to play. An important starting point is therefore sufficient knowledge of the law to be sure of the patient's rights. However, in the case study it is clear that Rose does need help and the nurse will not safeguard her patient by merely reminding her colleagues that they must act within the law. A more constructive approach is therefore needed. She may suggest giving Rose a little longer to adjust to a possible admission to hospital or explore other ways of assessing and treating Rose while keeping her at home.

Question 1.6

If a patient is not capable of taking full responsibility for her belongings, the hospital has to take this on board. Even if a patient is alert and capable, he should be advised of the risks of keeping valuables on the ward and an offer made to place these in the safekeeping of the hospital. If the patient does not wish to avail himself of this facility, the risk of theft or loss is his.

However, Rose's ability to care for her possessions is likely to be limited, and so the nurse may be wise to make a list of all items that Rose has with her. Certainly any valuables should be checked with another nurse, listed separately and a note made of any items locked away and of any jewellery left with Rose, for example, a wedding ring. Valuables will include jewellery, money, pension or cheque books and credit cards. Nurses must be careful of how they describe jewellery. Gold must be recorded as yellow metal, silver as white metal, and so on. This is to prevent false claims by patients.

Question 1.7

The Data Protection Act 1984 applies only to automatically processed data, i.e. material held on computer.

The Act contains certain principles, some of which Fiona would need to be aware of as she recorded confidential information on the computer terminal. She must have obtained the information lawfully and the amount of information must be adequate, relevant but not excessive for the purpose for which it is required. Thus Fiona should have some understanding of why the information is being transposed onto computer. The material collected must be accurate and up to date. Fiona's assessment and interviewing skills are important here. Confidential information must be protected against loss or disclosure. Fiona will have been given a special pass code to access information and she should ensure that the VDU (visual display unit) is not readily visible to visitors to the ward. Finally the data subject can request that any material about him is made available to him, but where medical information is involved, the doctor has the right to decide whether it is in the patient's interests to release this.

If Fiona fails to abide by the requirements of the Data Protection Act she can personally be taken to court for wrongful disclosure.

Question 1.8

If Rose left the ward there is a marked possibility of harm befalling her due to her poor physical and mental state but as already mentioned the legal powers of compulsorily keeping a patient in hospital are limited. The law does accept that in the short term, if a patient's 'right mind is not in him', it is necessary to detain a patient. This in conjunction with the duty of care the nurses owe to Rose to avoid negligent omissions means that the nurses acted appropriately and legally in preventing her leaving the ward.

Question 1.9

Restraining a patient could be seen as assault and battery by the nurses and therefore must only be used as a last resort to prevent harm resulting to the patient or others. The nurses might argue necessity in Rose's case, but the necessity appears to be in relation to getting on with their other work rather than to assist in Rose's treatment or care. Although it is possible to sympathize with the nurses' predicament, the conclusion has to be that the decision to restrain Rose has no legal base.

   Other methods of preventing Rose leaving the ward that are also realistic with staffing levels and the demands of other patients need to be explored. The nurses should ask both the doctor and the nurse manager for their advice.

Question 1.10

No, but it may be in the public interest or to the benefit of other members of the public to become involved. The decision is a moral or practical one.

Question 1.11

There is no compulsion to make statements to the police. However it may in the long term help to exonerate both herself and her colleagues by making statements rather than being afraid that such action might implicate her or her workmates.

   The following principles should be borne in mind. The statement must be accurate and factual, avoid assumptions and hearsay, be concise, clear and relevant while at the same time including sufficient detail of the situation being explored. It is always a good idea for the nurse to keep a copy of what she has written.

Question 1.12

In order to avoid a charge of assault and battery, it is legally necessary when treating or caring for a patient to gain his consent. However there are some patients who are incapable of giving a legally valid consent as this involves being able to understand what is being done. Rose is incapable of giving consent due to her confused state of mind, but the law accepts that in such circumstances if treatment is both urgent and necessary in order to save life or prevent grave illness or disability then it may be given. Thus the doctor and nurse are acting quite properly in the case study as long as the drugs given are those necessary for Rose's medical condition.

Question 1.13

No, the care plan is part of the nursing records about the patient. If the nurses did not even want to show the plan to the patient they would be acting quite legally. However, it is important that the patient cooperates with the care the nurses prescribe in order to benefit by it, so on practical grounds it is an excellent idea to involve the patient. If a care plan is drawn up that the patient feels he cannot go along with, he may become angry and frustrated. He may refuse to give his consent to nursing interventions or even discharge himself, a right that he has as long as he is not being legally detained in hospital. It is worth noting that under the Access to Health Records Act 1990 the patient can, at a later stage, apply for access to his health records although such a request can be refused.

Question 1.14

The doctor has overall responsibility for the patient and therefore takes the decision in discharging the patient from hospital. Hopefully he is helped in making such decisions by those professionals who have assisted in the care of the patient such as the nurses, occupational therapists and physiotherapists. The patient should be consulted but there is no legal requirement to do so and often he feels that few options are left to him. As mentioned above, a patient can discharge himself without medical agreement. In such circumstances he should be informed that such action is against medical advice and a written note made of what transpired. The patient may be asked to sign that he has understood the implications of self-discharge but cannot be made to do so.

Question 1.15

Home helps can be provided by the Local Authority under the Chronically Sick and Disabled Persons Act 1970. The Health Authority has a duty to provide a home nursing service under the NHS Act 1946.

Question 1.16

The nurses must check that the patient has received all her property on discharge. It is important to remember that bulky items such as a coat may have been stored away from the patient's bedside. Great care must also be taken to ensure that all valuables that have been handed over for safekeeping are returned and a receipt signed. Rose's initial property list will be useful to help check but it may well not be accurate as additional items may have been brought into hospital during Rose's stay and some taken home.

Question 1.17

This is not a question about the law! The answer has to be an ethical one, hinging on the professional's view of the importance of the individual being involved in making decisions about his own care. However, the law does give a framework in which both nurse and patient operate.

RELEVANT STATUTES

Access to Health Records Act 1990
Chronically Sick and Disabled Persons Act 1970
Data Protection Act 1984
Mental Health Act 1983
National Assistance Act 1948
National Assistance (Amendment) Act 1951
National Health Service Act 1946

REFERENCES

Medical Defence Union (1986) *Consent to Treatment*. Medical Defence Union, London.

National Consumer Council (1983) *Patients' Rights: a Guide for NHS patients and doctors*. HMSO, London.

Topliss, E. and Gould, B. (1981) *A Chapter for the Disabled*. Blackwell and Robertson, Oxford.

United Kingdom Central Council (1987) *Confidentiality, a UKCC Advisory Paper*. UKCC, London.

Young, A.P. (1989) *Legal Problems in Nursing Practice*, 2nd edn. Harper and Row, London.

2 Safety of patients and colleagues

At 48 years old, Charles Roberts is well satisfied with his life. He has a good job as an insurance assessor for a large company, a happy family with his second wife Olga and their two children, and a busy social life, bridge and wine tasting being particular interests. Although he smokes fairly heavily and is a bit overweight, he always feels fit and well. It is therefore a tremendous shock to the family when one evening after dinner he collapses and is rushed unconscious to the nearest casualty department.

The nurses carry out an assessment and document their findings which include the following:

Temperature: 36.5   Pulse: 70   Respiration: 20
Blood pressure: 160/100
Comments: Patient unconscious, responding to pain on left side only. Bruises on right arm and thigh.

Question 2.1   Why is the documentation of a patient's assessment legally so important?

Case Studies in Law and Nursing,
Ann P. Young.
Published in 1992 by
Chapman & Hall, London
ISBN 0 412 44130 6.

Activity 2.1
Look at the Accident and Emergency and ward assessment forms available to you. How clearly worded are they? How comprehensive?

Charles' wife has accompanied him, leaving a neighbour with the children. The doctor interviews Olga and says that he suspects that Olga's husband has had a stroke. In order to confirm this diagnosis, he urgently needs to order a brain scan. He asks Olga for her consent to this investigation.

Does the doctor need the wife's consent in these circumstances?   *Question 2.2*

This diagnosis is confirmed and Charles is admitted to a medical ward. After leaving her telephone number and asking to be informed of any change, his wife returns home. Frequent observations are continued through the night and by 6 am Charles has regained consciousness. However, his right side is paralyzed and he can only make gutteral noises. He is nursed in bed that day, his wife spending a large part of the day by his side while the children are at school. She asks to help wash and shave him so the nurses get a bowl of hot water for her and give strict instructions to call them when it comes to moving him. When Olga calls the nurses, she is looking angry and upset. She asks who has been mishandling her husband and points to the bruises on his right side. She says she does not expect her husband to be maltreated and she will find out who is responsible.

How can the nurses reassure Olga as well as preventing any unwanted legal action?   *Question 2.3*

During the next few days, Charles makes slow progress with a small amount of power returning to his right leg although his right arm remains totally useless. Amy, a staff nurse recently taking up employment in this hospital, is allocated to care for Charles on his third morning in hospital. She decides to sit him out of bed once he has had a wash, positions the chair by the bed and attempts to get Charles to stand and swivel with her support. However, Charles' weak leg gives way and he falls, pulling Amy with him: both end up on the floor. Several nurses rush to give assistance and after checking that Charles has no obvious injuries, lift him onto the chair. The nurse in charge informs the doctor and completes an accident form.

Question 2.4   Why must an accident form be completed?

The doctor examines Charles about 30 minutes later but can find no injuries. However, the nurses decide to reinstate more frequent neurological observations for the next two hours in case he hit his head as he fell.

Why is this decision by the nurses a sound one?

Activity 2.2
Because accidents to patients occur frequently, familiarize yourself
with the patient accident form in use in your health authority.

Amy continues to work for the remainder of the shift but by the time
she is due to go off duty, she tells the ward sister that her back is
getting increasingly painful from the accident with Charles. Sister is
annoyed with Amy for not saying anything sooner and asks her to fill
in an accident form for herself. Amy is unwilling to do so but the sister
gives her four reasons why it is advisable.

What are these four reasons?

The next day, the nursing officer for the medical unit receives a copy of
Amy's accident form and reads the following account of the incident:

> 'I was helping Mr Charles Roberts from the bed to the chair when
> he lost his balance and fell. In trying to support him, I hurt my back
> as he pulled me down. The pain in my back got worse so that it was
> very severe by the time I went off duty'.

The nursing officer feels that this description gives insufficient detail,
as well as potentially illustrating unsafe care.

Question 2.7   Can you identify the nursing officer's concerns?

Question 2.8   What legislation is particularly concerned with the safety of the workplace? How could this be applied in order to reduce the risk of nurses injuring their backs?

Unfortunately the nursing officer is unable to get clarification of Amy's statement as Amy is off sick with her injured back.

As Charles was hypertensive on admission, he has been prescribed daily drugs to lower his blood pressure and therefore reduce the risk of a further stroke. Two days after his fall, Charles is sitting out of bed watching the evening television programmes with some other patients. Two nurses bring the 6 pm drugs around and give Charles his anti-hypertensive drug. Too late they realize that he has only been pre-scribed the drug for 7 am, this dose having been given at the time stated.

What can the nurses do to reduce the risk of negligence following this error?   *Question 2.9*

Fortunately Charles comes to no harm following this error, but the following day the two nurses are interviewed by the nursing officer and warned that such mistakes are unacceptable and must not be repeated. The nursing officer's action is based on the health authority's drug and disciplinary policies.

Activity 2.3
Find out where your local drug and disciplinary policies are kept. You will certainly need to become familiar with the drug policy so read this carefully.

Why are these policies important in promoting safe care?   *Question 2.10*

For the first few days of his admission, Charles' care plan is amended daily but once his progress slows, the care plan is reviewed weekly and amended if necessary. However his care is evaluated daily.

Question 2.11 What is the legal requirement for the frequency of documenting patient care?

Part of Charles' care plan and evaluation of care after three weeks is shown below:

Date	Problem	Goal	Plan	Signature	Date Evaluation	Signature
9.2.92	Reduced mobility due to CVA	To encourage independence within his limits.	To stand with support and walk a few steps with two nurses.		Managed to walk from bed to bathroom but chair back. Care given.	
		To prevent possible complications of immobility such as pressure sores and chest infection.	To move position 2 hourly. Physio to chest daily.		Care given. Care given.	

Question 2.12 What would make this record a more useful document in case of any legal action?

Activity 2.4
Look at some of the patient care plans available to you. Do they fulfil the legal requirements suggested?

One morning Charles indicates that he would like to go to the day room for a cigarette. By now he is walking with the assistance of a nurse and a tripod. The nurse settles Charles in a chair and lights a cigarette for him. As it is a busy morning, she asks him if he will be alright and then returns to her other patients.

Is she acting correctly in leaving Charles to smoke on his own?

Question 2.13

Throughout the period of his hospitalization, Olga visits daily and brings the children, who are 10 and 7 years old, with her at weekends. One Saturday afternoon, the nurse in charge notices that the younger child looks very flushed and has a fine red rash on her face that looks like measles. The nurse points this out to Olga, who admits that there have been some children with measles at school. The nurse is angry that Olga has risked the health of the patients by letting the child visit and asks her to leave with the children.

Does the nurse have the legal authority to require visitors to leave the ward?

Question 2.14

Activity 2.5

Find out what rules your health authority has about visitors, particularly children.

A week later one of the ward nurses contracts measles and phones in sick. She is very well aware of the risk her infection would present to already ill and debilitated patients. She has a clear duty to protect her patients from hazards even when this means leaving the ward short staffed.

Activity 2.6
What regulations does your Occupational Health Department have regarding nurses who pose an infection risk to patients?

After a further 4 weeks, Charles is mobilizing with a tripod only and the nurses are encouraging him to go for walks on his own. Another patient comes to tell one of the nurses that Charles has fallen over in the toilet. Charles seems more angry than shaken but the usual checks are made for any injuries and an accident form is completed.

Question 2.15   Have the nurses been negligent in allowing Charles to walk about unattended when he is still a bit unsteady on his feet?

Soon after this episode, plans are made for Charles to return home. Initially a weekend visit is to be attempted. This is of limited success, as Charles has difficulty in manoeuvring in the bathroom and toilet. The occupational therapist suggests a bath seat and handrail in the bathroom and a handrail in the toilet.

Question 2.16   Is there any statutory help for the provision of such aids?

Three months after admission Charles returns home. He is to continue speech therapy and physiotherapy on an outpatient basis. Charles' employers have been concerned and supportive during his illness but as it seems less and less likely that Charles will regain full use of his right arm or verbal fluency, after a further 3 months he is dismissed from his job.

Are his employers acting legally?

Question 2.17

Charles makes some further small improvements and he and his family adapt to his disabilities.

ANSWERS

Question 2.1

There is always the possibility of a patient taking legal action of some kind against a nurse or a health authority even if there are no good grounds for this. The most likely action is to sue for negligence but the patient may also bring a complaint against the hospital or, in a private establishment, sue additionally for breach of contract. In all cases, there may well be a time lapse before the patient takes legal action, usually up to three years for negligence, one year for bringing a complaint and six years for breach of contract. These examples illustrate the importance of an accurate and comprehensive written assessment which is a yardstick against which to measure the patient's condition at a later stage of treatment and acts as a permanent record long after the nurse's memory of that particular patient has faded.

Question 2.2

Nobody can give consent to treatment for another adult and therefore it is legally quite unnecessary for the doctor to ask Olga for her consent. Charles is, of course, incapable of giving consent, but the doctor can proceed with any investigations and treatment on the basis that they are so urgent and necessary that Charles would have given his consent if he had been able to do so. It would also be likely that not to take such action could be considered negligent if the patient suffered further harm due to this omission.

In spite of there being no legal basis for obtaining a relative's consent, nurses will often see such action taken. It seems that doctors sometimes want to 'play safe' and reduce the possibility of later litigation by acting in this way.

Question 2.3

This question illustrates the importance of a careful and comprehensive initial assessment. By explaining that the bruises were noted on admission, the chance of any successful legal action is ruled out. However, the nurses could go further by suggesting that perhaps her husband sustained bruising as he collapsed with the stroke, thus underlining the likelihood that no one is to blame.

Question 2.4

There is always the possibility that an accident could have been avoidable and therefore potential negligence on the part of the nurses caring for the patient.

At this point it is worth exploring what is meant legally by negligence. First the nurse has to have a 'duty of care' towards the patient. Amy seems clearly to have this duty as she is working on the ward and in addition has been allocated to care for Charles. Second there must be some failure in the performance of that duty, either by act or omission. This seems less clear from the case study. The standard of care given must be that expected of an ordinary nurse in that speciality, so if Amy was correctly using a technique accepted as satisfactory for moving a partially paralyzed patient, then she did not fail in her duty. However, if, considering the circumstances, she had not chosen the most suitable technique or carried it out wrongly, then she would have failed to reach the standard expected. Finally for negligence to succeed in court, the patient must have suffered harm as a result of the nurse's failure – hence the legal importance of checking if Charles has any injuries.

As illustrated in questions 2.1 and 2.3, good documentation protects nurses from unnecessary litigation and a written record is vital because of the lapse of time before legal action is taken.

Question 2.5

Practically, any head injury needs prompt detection for satisfactory treatment to be undertaken. Legally, if the neurological observations show no cerebral damage subsequent to the accident, any later possible deterioration of Charles' condition cannot be blamed on his fall.

Question 2.6

1. To ensure Amy receives a medical check and she is given the proper treatment and advice.
2. In case Amy has to have prolonged time off work, she can claim benefits under Industrial Injuries Benefit from the DSS if there is evidence of an injury at work.
3. In case Amy has to give up nursing and wants to see if she has grounds for suing the health authority for damages.

4. To enable the health authority to monitor the incidence of back injuries amongst nurses and to take any action necessary to reduce these.

Question 2.7

Amy has failed to state *how* she was assisting the patient to move. It is therefore impossible to assess potential negligence as explained in question 2.4. Amy also states that she hurt her back in trying to support Charles. It was foolish of Amy to act in this way. All nurses must be aware of how back injuries occur and that it is much better to let the patient fall in a controlled way than to risk back injury by trying to keep the patient standing. It would also have been helpful if Amy had stated why she was attempting to move the patient on her own instead of getting assistance.

Question 2.8

Two areas of legislation are important. The law on negligence places a general duty of care on the employer to take steps to prevent injuries to staff. More specifically the Health and Safety at Work (etc.) Act 1974, requires positive steps by both employer and employee to promote safety in the workplace.

In relation to back injuries, the employer responsibility is as follows:

1. To provide adequate training in lifting and moving patients. Sufficient training must be given to ensure the safety of nurse, patient and her colleagues and it is important that regular updating is given, particularly when new members of staff take up employment (as in Amy's case).
2. To ensure that there are adequate staff to cope with the physical demands of lifting and moving patients. However in a non-emergency situation, the employer is likely to argue that a nurse can wait for assistance if necessary.
3. To provide proper tools and a safe system of working. Hoists, slings and other equipment must be supplied and maintained. Ward layout should be such that it is possible to use the equipment and to lift safely.

The employee also has duties under the Act. She must take reasonable care of her own health and safety and that of others who may be affected by her actions. Thus Amy has a responsibility to protect both herself and her patients from injury. She must also cooperate with others to promote safety and this will involve attendance at training sessions offered and use of equipment supplied.

Question 2.9

For negligence to occur, the patient must suffer harm as a result of the nurses' actions. Therefore it is important that they inform the doctor of their error and monitor the patient's condition for any adverse effects. If there are signs of overdosage then an antidote can be given.

Question 2.10

A policy, although not binding in the same way as the law, has to be followed if the nurse is to avoid repercussions on her employment position. The ultimate action against a nurse for failing to abide by a policy would be dismissal if her action was serious enough to be considered gross misconduct or if less serious breaches of policy were repeated on several occasions.

The drug policy therefore requires nurses to follow certain rules when administering drugs. These rules have been decided after consultation and discussion between representatives of management and workers on what constitutes safe practice. The disciplinary policy draws up regulations to be followed when discipline of a member of staff becomes necessary and it operates within the wider remit of the Employment Protection (Consolidation) Act 1978. Discipline is important in maintaining standards, not just to point out when an employee has failed to act properly, but also to assist that employee to improve her performance.

Question 2.11

Care should be documented whenever there is a change, any untoward occurrence, an omission of care or when a review date has been set. The frequency of documenting care may therefore quite legitimately vary greatly depending on the condition of the patient. The decisions regarding Charles' nursing records seem reasonable.

Question 2.12

1. The problem is very vaguely worded. Reduced mobility means very little and it is not stated which side of the body is weak.
2. Abbreviations should be avoided unless very common and understood by all nurses.
3. The goals are nurse centred rather than patient centred but still give a reasonably clear picture.
4. The plan is rather sketchy and legally should contain more detail.
5. The fact that the planned care has been given fails to state whether this was adequate to maintain the patient's condition. The first part of the evaluation is better as it gives proper feedback on the patient's response to care.
6. Date and full signature are vital in case of later legal action, both to pinpoint events and to trace potential witnesses.

Question 2.13

This depends on whether she has checked, then or on a previous occasion, that Charles can hold the cigarette securely and has an ashtray that he can reach. If she has not satisfied herself as to his safety, she could be negligent if Charles dropped the cigarette and burnt himself or set the furnishings alight.

Question 2.14

Yes. The hospital is Crown property, not public property and visitors can only stay at the discretion of the staff. Once asked to leave, they become trespassers if they fail to do so and can be evicted. Usual practice would be for the nurse in charge or the nursing officer to initiate such action.

Question 2.15

This is a complex issue for both the legal and nursing professions. In many situations, nurses have to make decisions that involve some degree of risk. In fact the law on negligence can assist rather than hinder such decision making in the following way.

In planning Charles' care the nurses need to weigh up the good versus the harm of allowing Charles more freedom. The harm is clearly that Charles falls and injures himself, the good is that he regains confidence and independence. They need to consider the risks of *not* allowing him freedom, the harm of keeping him dependent and suffering the damaging effects of immobility versus the good of preventing accidental damage. If on balance, the good of allowing Charles freedom and the harm of not allowing him independence outweigh the opposite argument, then the nurses will not be negligent in taking that risk. In fact, they could be negligent in taking the opposite action. The law will also consider what is accepted practice, and this also supports encouraging rehabilitation. Finally, the nurses need to weigh up the likelihood of various outcomes. These may vary with different patients in similar circumstances and with the same patient at different times. The nurses need to show that they have acted reasonably in reaching a decision.

Question 2.16

Yes. Under the Chronically Sick and Disabled Persons Act 1970, local authorities must make arrangements to meet the particular needs of the disabled, including giving assistance in works of adaptation. However, the local authority has discretion on the criteria to use in identifying need and this leads to patchy application of the law.

Question 2.17

A legal reason for dismissal is incapability and long-term sickness clearly comes into this category. Charles' employment contract is likely to state rights regarding notice to be given. His employers appear to have been generous in the amount of time elapsing before dismissal finally took place.

RELEVANT STATUTES

Chronically Sick and Disabled Persons Act 1970
Criminal Justice Act 1988
Employment Protection (Consolidation) Act 1978
Health and Safety at Work (etc.) Act 1974

REFERENCES

Beckett, A. and Young, A. (1989) *Health and Safety at Work in Checks and Balances*. Diploma in Nursing, Distance Learning Centre, South Bank Polytechnic, London.

Capper, A. (1989) *Employment Legislation in Checks and Balances*. Diploma in Nursing, Distance Learning Centre, South Bank Polytechnic, London.

Carson, D. and Montgomery, J. (1989) *Nursing and the Law*. Macmillan Education, London.

Cowan, V. (1987) *Documentation Nursing* (Oxford) Vol. 3(14), p. 527.

Rogers, R. and Salvage, J. (1988) *Nurses at Risk*. Heinemann Nursing, Oxford.

Communicating with patients, relatives and colleagues

3

At 2 pm one Sunday afternoon, the police bring a middle-aged woman to the Accident and Emergency Department. She is wearing a stained skirt, a jumper with holes in it, no stockings and canvas shoes. She has no coat although it is cool outdoors and no other property or valuables. The police explain that they found her walking erratically along the road, hurling abuse at the car drivers. When the police tried to reason with her, she threw grit and dirt at them. They decided that she was acting in a way that was a danger both to herself and to others and that they had no choice but to bring her to the hospital.

On what legal grounds are the police acting?

Question 3.1

The nurses on duty carry out an initial assessment. Shakira, a registered general nurse, notes that the woman smells of alcohol. She is critical of the police for bringing in an 'old methie' and wasting their time. Why not show her out? Her colleague, Mary, is less sure.

Can a person presenting to the Accident and Emergency Department be refused treatment?

Question 3.2

Case Studies in Law and Nursing,
Ann P. Young.
Published in 1992 by
Chapman & Hall, London
ISBN 0 412 44130 6.

Shakira and Mary try to get some information from the woman without success. She will not give them her name, accuses them of acting for the devil and says that God has told her to destroy all devil worshippers. The two nurses are unsure what to record and seek help from the sister in charge. However, like Shakira and Mary, she is only general, and not mental, trained.

Question 3.3

Have Shakira and Mary acted appropriately in seeking help from the sister?

The sister suggests Shakira and Mary continue with their assessment, and take a baseline set of observations of pulse, temperature and blood pressure. As they attempt to do this, the woman pushes them away and makes for the exit door.

Question 3.4

Should the nurses prevent her from leaving?

The woman is persuaded to return and shortly after this the doctor arrives to examine her. He decides that she is mentally ill and suggests to the woman that she be admitted to the psychiatric unit. At this she becomes very abusive so that the doctor feels that the only option is to place her under a Section of the Mental Health Act.

Question 3.5

Which Section of the Mental Health Act 1983 would be used?

Activity 3.1

Make a list of the possible formal admissions under the Mental Health Act 1983.

The doctor telephones the duty psychiatrist who arranges the woman's admission. In the meantime as she is so restless she is prescribed a

sedative to be given by intramuscular injection. This is then given.
    The woman is transferred to a psychiatric ward 45 minutes later.
Mary accompanies her and hands her over to the ward nurse.

For legal reasons, what information should be given to the ward nurse?

Question 3.6

The woman remains drowsy for the rest of the day and sedation is again administered at 10 pm although she is no longer abusive or restless.

Is it justifiable to continue to sedate this patient?

Question 3.7

The next morning the woman appears to be more alert and less affected by her delusions. She says her name is Deirdre Maloney. The police are informed and come back with the information that she has had inpatient treatment elsewhere due to a long history of mental illness. They promise to contact the ward again once they have more information. The nurse in charge contacts the administrators at this hospital and asks if Deirdre's notes could be sent to them. The answer to this request is 'no'.

Why was the request refused? What would have been a more effective way of getting the information required?

Question 3.8

Staff nurse Harry Lyme is allocated to care for Deirdre. The first thing he does is to sit and talk with her. Once he feels he has made contact with her he explains about her admission under Section and her legal rights under the Mental Health Act. He then gives her a leaflet entitled *Your rights under the Mental Health Act 1983*.

Activity 3.2

Find out what information should have been given to Deirdre. Get a copy of the leaflet and read it carefully.

Harry then plans Deirdre's care for the day. A student nurse, Rhoda McDonald who has been on the ward for two weeks, is being supervized by Harry so he decides to delegate some of Deirdre's care to her. He suggests that Rhoda assists Deirdre with her hygiene needs. Rhoda introduces herself and tells Deirdre that she is to come and have a bath. Deirdre refuses, but Rhoda insists at which point Deirdre becomes very angry and abusive. Harry returns to the scene to find out what all the shouting is about. He sends the student to do another job while he calms Deirdre and suggests that a wash at the washbasin may be sufficient today. However, Deirdre accuses him of being the devil, so he withdraws from the situation for the time being.

Question 3.9   It appears that the student has possibly worsened Deirdre's mental state by her approach. However, it was Harry who asked Rhoda to care for Deirdre without being specific in his instructions. Was Harry wrong in the way he delegated this care?

Are there any circumstances where it is not appropriate to give a patient choice as regards personal cleanliness? *Question 3.10*

Harry finds Rhoda in tears in the office. He tells her that she acted wrongly and she should have known better. Rhoda asks if this incident will affect her ward assessment.

What legal responsibilities do the trained staff have regarding the assessment of student nurses? *Question 3.11*

Activity 3.3
Check your own practical assessment procedures for the rights of both assessors and students.

Later that day Deirdre is seen by the doctor and a drug regime prescribed. The nurses give Deirdre her medication straight away. On Deirdre asking what the pills are for, the nurse says they are vitamin pills and the patient then swallows them.

Is it legally ever justifiable to lie to a patient about his/her treatment? *Question 3.12*

Activity 3.4
Read the UKCC leaflet on *Exercising Accountability* Section D Consent and Truth, pp. 10–11.

The police telephone the ward that evening to give the name and address of a next of kin, a sister, Miss Bridget Maloney who lives five miles away. They have already contacted her to tell her that Deirdre is in hospital.

After 72 hours, the Section Order holding Deirdre in hospital as a formal patient expires. A conference between the psychiatrist, a social worker allocated to Deirdre and the ward nurse is held.

Question 3.13   What are the legal responsibilities of each of these people towards Deirdre?

The nurses suggest that Deirdre now seems amenable to treatment so the psychiatrist decides to let Deirdre continue with treatment as an informal patient.

Question 3.14   In these circumstances, could Deirdre be forced to have treatment against her will?

Over the next two weeks Deirdre's condition shows improvement although she continues to have some delusional thoughts. The nurses feel that some adjustment is needed to the drug regime and suggest this to the doctor.

Are the nurses acting properly in making such a suggestion?   *Question 3.15*

Activity 3.5

Read the UKCC leaflet on *Administration of Medicines* The Framework, pp. 5–10.

Bridget Maloney, Deirdre's sister, makes contact with the ward, initially by telephone. The nurse who answers the telephone explains to the caller why Deirdre has been admitted to hospital and a brief description of the treatment.

What information should be given to a relative over the telephone?   *Question 3.16*

Bridget Maloney later visits her sister. After Deirdre has been in hospital for four weeks, the doctor suggests that Deirdre be discharged home to the care of Bridget for a while. Deirdre could hopefully pick up the threads of her life with some support. Bridget agrees to the suggestion but says it will take her a week to get her flat organized.

The following day the doctor discharges Deirdre as her bed is urgently needed for another patient.

Question 3.17   Does the doctor have the right to discharge a patient against the patient's or her relatives' wishes?

Rather unwillingly, Bridget collects her sister and takes her home. The ward staff apologize and, although feeling very embarrassed, put the incident to one side. One week later, the hospital administrator informs them that he has received a letter of complaint from Miss Bridget Maloney regarding the failure of the hospital to give her proper notice of her sister's discharge.

Question 3.18   How should this complaint be dealt with?

Activity 3.6
Look up your own health authority's complaints policy.

After the complaint has been investigated, the hospital apologizes to Bridget Maloney and brings to the attention of its staff the importance of careful discharge planning.

ANSWERS

Question 3.1

Under the Mental Health Act 1983 (Section 136), a police constable finding a person in a public place who appears to be suffering from a mental disorder and in immediate need of care or control can take this person to a 'place of safety'. This is defined in the Act as a police station, a psychiatric hospital, a mental nursing home or local authority residential accommodation for the mentally disordered.

Question 3.2

No. The principle of the Accident and Emergency Department is that anyone seeking treatment should be seen. The staff could be negligent if they turned somebody away without properly assessing him if he then suffered harm because of a failure to treat.

Question 3.3

The two nurses very rightly recognized the limitations of their competence and took action to remedy the situation by seeking help. In this way they reduced any risk of negligence due to their own lack of skill or knowledge. It is also likely that if anything had been missed in the patient's assessment, the sister would have been liable, being in a position of authority over the other nurses. The fact that she also was only general trained does not remove the responsibility from her.

Question 3.4

Yes. The police have reported that she has been acting in a way that is a danger both to herself and to others. In addition to any considerations under the Mental Health Act, the nurses could be failing in their duty towards her if they let her go and could be negligent if harm then resulted.

Question 3.5

Section 4 Emergency admission for assessment, valid for 72 hours.

Question 3.6

1. The woman should be identified in some way and this must be pointed out to the ward nurse. A hospital number may be all that can be used at present.

2. Property must be checked by the two nurses against the property list made in the Accident and Emergency Department.
3. The fact that sedation has been given, what and when, so that her safety can be maintained as she gets drowsy.
4. The fact that alcohol may also be a factor in case the woman suffers the effects of alcohol poisoning or is alcoholic.
5. The involvement of the police as they are likely to follow up on their initial intervention. Their names and police station would also be useful information.

Question 3.7

As the patient is under Section, it is justifiable to give certain treatment, even without the patient's consent, if it is immediately necessary to:

1. save the patient's life or
2. prevent a serious deterioration of her condition (the treatment not being irreversible) or
3. alleviate serious suffering by the patient (the treatment not being irreversible or hazardous)
4. and represents the minimum interference necessary to prevent the patient from behaving violently or being a danger to herself or others.

Giving a sedative is certainly not irreversible and probably not hazardous although that would be a medical decision, so the third point probably applies. The last point may well also apply – again the decision as to what would be the minimal drug dosage in these circumstances would have to be a medical one. How immediately necessary is a second administration of sedative seems more debatable but again on legal grounds the nurse can accept the doctor's decision.

Question 3.8

Medical notes are owned by the health authority in which the patient has been treated while the information within them is controlled by the medical practitioner who was in charge of the patient. There is no compulsion to release these notes to anyone other than the patient concerned unless required to do so by a court of law.

The nurse in charge should have considered what information she wanted regarding the *nursing* of this patient but any response would still be at the discretion of the other hospital's administrators, bearing in mind confidentiality aspects. Any medical information must be requested by the doctor responsible for the patient.

Question 3.9

In order to delegate safely, the person receiving the delegated task must be competent to carry it out.

For Harry to be confident that he is acting properly in delegating care to Rhoda, he would need to have assured himself of her skill in dealing with this type of situation. He could have done this by:

1. having observed her with other patients with similar problems;
2. asking her how she would go about planning Deirdre's hygiene needs;
3. staying with her to observe her skill in this situation.

As Rhoda is a student nurse Harry really cannot assume she has the appropriate skills without checking in one of the ways listed above. If the patient suffered harm because of Rhoda's incompetence, he would be negligent in delegation.

Rhoda would also be responsible for any negligence towards the patient in spite of being unqualified. She therefore has a responsibility for ensuring that trained staff realize her limitations. Unfortunately inexperience can sometimes make it difficult for the student to appreciate her lack of skill.

Question 3.10

A patient cannot be forced to take a bath against his will! However, if the state of hygiene of a patient is so poor as to constitute a risk to the health of other patients, for example due to infection, infestation or obnoxious smell, he could be given the option of bathing or being discharged from hospital. Obviously this is an extreme measure and most patients are willing to cooperate with hospital staff to some extent if dealt with tactfully.

The situation with a mentally ill patient under Section is a little more complicated as the hospital may be negligent if discharging him too soon before treatment has had an effect. On the other hand, the dangers of an unwashed patient are physically less on a psychiatric ward than a general ward with debilitated patients. The bath can wait a few days!

Question 3.11

The assessor has a responsibility towards the patients that reasonable care is given by the student. Therefore a failure to assess properly or to act appropriately where performance is poor could be negligence.

The assessor has a duty to inform the student of any adverse assessment and to offer help to improve. A legal responsibility under employment legislation is to be fair to an employee where discipline or dismissal is a possibility. Although the student undertaking Project 2000 training does not fall into this category, the same rules of good practice are likely to be applied.

Any documentation must be signed and dated by the assessor as potential legal documents.

Question 3.12

No. A patient normally has to consent to treatment and to do so has to understand the implications of this. However, there is no legal necessity to give a full explanation although many nurses would feel that the more information patients receive, the better are they able to cooperate with care. In addition, if a patient asks for information regarding treatment, normally the legal duty to answer such questions is increased.

The case may be put forward that to tell the patient what the pills are for could cause Deirdre psychological harm although this seems unlikely. The choice might then be to give limited information, for example, 'the pills are to make you feel better'. Any further questions of Deirdre's could be referred to a senior nurse or the doctor if there was concern as to Deirdre's possible reaction.

Therefore on legal grounds there is no justification for lying.

Question 3.13

The doctor has overall responsibility for the patient. He controls admission, discharge and prescription of treatment. The Mental Health Act also has clearly specified medical duties for formal detention of patients under the Act.

The social worker will be approved to take on special responsibilities with the mentally ill after additional training. Under the Mental Health Act 1983 he/she can also be involved in formal admissions and aftercare of patients.

The nurse has a responsibility to carry out treatment prescribed by the doctor. The Mental Health Act 1983 specifies that where psychosurgery or electroconvulsive therapy is proposed, there may be a legal duty to consult the nurse. For other nursing care, there is a legal duty under the law on negligence to give care of a standard expected of a reasonable nurse in similar circumstances.

Question 3.14

No. An informal patient gives consent to treatment in exactly the same way as someone who is not mentally ill. However, if her condition deteriorated and she then refused treatment, the psychiatrist might consider it necessary to put her back on Section (Section 5) when treatment for the mental disorder could be given without consent.

Question 3.15

Yes. As stated in question 3.13, the doctor is responsible for prescribing treatment but the nurses will be monitoring the effect of any medication on the patient as part of their duties. They therefore have a responsibility to report to the doctor the patient's progress so that he can adjust care accordingly. A doctor often appreciates the experienced nurse making suggestions regarding medication.

The area of the nurse's involvement with drug prescribing is one that is changing rapidly at present. Particularly in the community nurses who have undergone extra training are being given the responsibility of modifying drug prescriptions within certain well-defined limits. Such change carries important legal implications regarding the extension of the nurse's role and must not be taken on without the approval of the nurse's employer.

Question 3.16

Unless the caller is well known to the ward staff, the answer to this is minimal information only. The enquiry could be fraudulent or the ramifications within families can be complex so that it may be difficult for the nurse to be sure to whom she is talking. For example, the caller may only identify herself as a 'sister'. There is also the question of breach of confidentiality.

In Deirdre's case, it would have been preferable to have confirmed that she was on the ward and that she was making some progress, then to suggest the caller visits when arrangements can be made to discuss the situation in more depth.

Question 3.17

Yes. The doctor has the legal right to decide when to discharge a patient. If this discharge is later found to have been too early on medical grounds resulting in a deterioration of the patient's condition, negligence could exist. From the practical point of view, social reasons for delaying discharge rarely carry legal weight although very often being a major concern to the patient and relatives. However, community nurses can veto patient discharges from psychiatric units if they feel community services cannot support them. Unfortunately the doctor is often caught between conflicting demands.

Question 3.18

The Hospital Complaints Procedure Act 1985 requires that complaints must be dealt with in the following way.

1. An officer is designated to receive written complaints which should be made within six months of the incident.
2. This officer should be of sufficient seniority to command the confidence of patients and relatives and the cooperation of the staff concerned.
3. Response to the complaint should be thorough, fair and speedy.
4. Any staff implicated should be given the opportunity to reply.
5. All those involved should be kept fully informed of the progress of the investigation.
6. If the complainant is not satisfied with the conduct or outcome of the hospital's investigation, he/she can take the complaint to the Health Service Commissioner. He has a duty to investigate complaints where

injustice or hardship has resulted because of a failure in the service or because of maladministration. He cannot act if the complaint is the subject of a court case or involves clinical judgement.

7. If a complaint is upheld, an apology should be sent to the complainant. Action should be taken to ensure that such a situation does not recur but this cannot be legally enforced. The Health Service Commissioner publishes a report every six months of the complaints investigated by his office.

RELEVANT STATUTES AND CASES

Employment Protection (Consolidation) Act 1978
Hospital Complaints Procedure Act 1985
Mental Health Act 1983
Barnett *v.* Chelsea and Kensington H.M.C. 1969
Sidaway *v.* Board of Governors of the Bethlem Royal and Maudsley Hospital 1984

REFERENCES

Brazier, M. (1987) *Medicine, Patients and the Law*. Penguin, Harmondsworth, Middlesex.

Department of Health (1989) Discharge of Patients from Hospital. Hc(89)5. HMSO, London.

Department of Health and Welsh Office (1990) *Code of Practice*. Mental Health Act 1983, HMSO, London.

United Kingdom Central Council (1986) *Administration of Medicines*, a UKCC Advisory Paper. UKCC, London.

United Kingdom Central Council (1989) *Exercising Accountability*, a UKCC Advisory Document. UKCC, London.

Young, A.P. (1989) *Legal Problems in Nursing Practice*, 2nd edn. Harper and Row, London.

Working in the community

4

Mary Chin has been working as a district nurse for the last 18 months in an inner city area. Most of her patients are from lower socio-economic groups with problems of poor housing and unemployment or low paid jobs. There is also quite a high proportion of elderly people in her area. Mary enjoys her work and finds it particularly rewarding to work with the whole family. She is impressed at the strength and determination that most families under pressure display towards their members. Today she is going to spend part of the morning with one such family.

Joe has multiple sclerosis. At 40 years old, the disease is already far advanced and he can only get around in a wheelchair. As the family live in a second floor flat it is difficult for Joe to get out, and impossible if the lift has been vandalized. Mary arrives at about 9.30 am, letting herself in with the key the family has given her as Joe's wife will be out at work.

In accepting the key, has the nurse acted properly in the circumstances?

Question 4.1

Joe's daughter Lara, is at home today. She says she is taking the day off sick from work. Mary greets Joe who seems rather depressed in spite of being out yesterday with a neighbour. He explains that there was nothing but 'hassle'. He had wanted to choose a birthday card for his wife but could not get into the first two shops he tried because of steps.

Case Studies in Law and Nursing,
Ann P. Young.
Published in 1992 by
Chapman & Hall, London
ISBN 0 412 44130 6.

Question 4.2   What help must be provided for the disabled regarding access to buildings?

Activity 4.1
Walk round your local shopping centre and check the access allowed to people in wheelchairs.

Joe then visited the council offices to find out if there was any chance of being rehoused in a ground floor flat.

Question 4.3   What help is the disabled person legally entitled to with regard to housing?

Mary, while being sympathetic, makes sure that Joe understands both his rights under the law and its limitations. She admires the card that Joe eventually managed to buy and then suggests a bath. Joe is very keen but breaks the news to Mary that the hoist has been broken for the last week. However, he is sure that Lara will help Mary lift him into the bath.

Is Joe responsible for ensuring that the hoist is in working order?   *Question 4.4*

Activity 4.2
Find out who provides and maintains equipment in patients' homes.

Lara agrees to help so Mary decides to proceed with Joe's bath.

Could Mary have refused to bath Joe?   *Question 4.5*

Mary and Lara get Joe into the bath without difficulty but when lifting him out Mary strains her back as Lara fails to position herself correctly, leaving Mary with most of Joe's weight.

What should Mary do in these circumstances in order to protect herself?   *Question 4.6*

Once Joe is comfortably settled with a cup of tea, he reverts to talking about the limitations imposed on him by his condition. He says he feels helpless but there is nothing wrong with his brain. He also feels guilty because his wife has to do dirty and poorly paid jobs, mostly cleaning, and he wishes he could help. Is there something he could do? His arms are weak but he could still use his hands.

Question 4.7   What employment rights do the disabled have?

Activity 4.3
Find out how many disabled people are employed in your health authority. What jobs do they do?

Mary promises to contact Joe's social worker and ask him/her to give Joe some advice.

As Mary leaves, Lara comes to the door with her and asks for a quick word. She tells Mary she is pregnant but her parents do not know yet. She asks Mary what she should do but Mary tells her only she can make the decision as to whether she wants to have the baby or not.

Question 4.8   What are the legal grounds for abortion?

Lara thinks she may keep the baby but she is worried about money
even though she has a reasonable job which she has held for just over
a year.

What rights will Lara be entitled to if she decides to ask for maternity
leave?

Question 4.9

Mary asks Lara what she will do about the baby if she goes back to
work. Lara has a friend who went to a child minder but she was rather
expensive and a creche might be cheaper.

How could Lara learn about local child minding facilities?

Question 4.10

> **Activity 4.4**
> Find out if your health authority has a creche and what the charges are.

As Mary is driving to her next appointment, she passes a group of people standing over someone lying on the pavement.

Question 4.11   Should Mary stop and investigate?

Mary pulls up and goes to see what assistance she can give. She is told that an ambulance has been called. On assessing the patient, she finds he is unconscious but still breathing. She asks one of the bystanders to help her roll him onto his side so that his airway can be maintained. Belatedly she notices that the leg onto which he has been rolled is probably broken as it is no longer aligned properly.

Question 4.12   Could Mary be in legal diffculties because of her actions?

The ambulance arrives within a few minutes and Mary continues on her way to her next patient, an elderly lady with leg ulcers that need redressing. When she arrives there is no answer to the doorbell so Mary has to return to the health centre without seeing her.

Question 4.13   Why is it important that Mary documents that she has visited this lady's house but not seen her?

There is a team meeting at the health centre at lunch time so Mary meets her colleagues and exchanges news with them. As they cover each other's patients on days off, sickness and holidays, they have to work closely together. The main topic of discussion for this meeting is increasing workloads due to ever earlier discharge from hospital of patients who are still unwell or incapacitated. Peter, a nurse not yet qualified as a district nurse, is particularly concerned at the difficulties he faces in maintaining standards under these conditions and worries that patients will suffer as a result.

What advice can be given to Peter to help him avoid possible negligence?

Question 4.14

Another nurse, Diana, says angrily that there is a limit to how much they can take on. Patients should not be discharged so early.

Can the nursing officer produce a sound legal argument to support this?

Question 4.15

After lunch Mary has several more visits to make in a tower block on her patch. She does not like going to this block as only two weeks ago another nurse was mugged and robbed there.

Question 4.16   List some of the precautions that Mary could take to protect herself.

Activity 4.5
Find out what advice the police give to community nurses.

Mary organizes for a colleague to accompany her although this further increases their workload. However, Mary has told her nursing officer that she will not go to the block on her own.

Question 4.17   What are the responsibilities of the health authority in these circumstances?

Question 4.18   Can Mary refuse to visit the patients in this block?

Mary's first visit is to a young woman, Carmel, who has two young children. She has recently had a gynaecological operation and the abdominal wound has partially broken down since her discharge home. While Mary is dressing the wound, the two year old comes to sit with her mother. Mary notices that the child has a bad bruise on the side of her face and asks Carmel about this. Carmel quickly explains that the child fell over while playing outside. Mary feels dubious but decides to say nothing further.

What legislation could be involved if Mary suspected that the child was the victim of abuse?

Question 4.19

Mary is in the process of clearing up when Carmel's husband comes in. He appears to have been drinking, swears at Mary and her colleague and tells them to get out. Mary quietly says they are just leaving and quickly picks up her bag.

How could Mary go about planning any future visits to this home?

Question 4.20

Mary and her colleague complete their afternoon visits without further trouble and return to the health centre. There Mary completes any documentation of care that is outstanding before going home.

Activity 4.6
Compare the community and hospital nursing documents available to you. Look for similarities as well as differences.

ANSWERS

Question 4.1

It is dubious practice for a nurse to accept the patient's front door key. Firstly, if the nurse entered the property when the patient was not in she could be accused of trespassing. Secondly, if there was a theft from the flat, she would have to account for her whereabouts and the security of the key. Both situations could lead to unpleasantness at the least, legal action at the worst.

However, the question of access is important to both disabled patient and nurse. A patient must be dissuaded from leaving a key under a mat or on a length of string inside the letter box as such measures are easily discovered by thieves. Probably the most satisfactory answer is for the patient to leave the key with a trusted neighbour. The nurse can then collect it from and return it to this person.

Question 4.2

The answer to this may well be, none. Section 4 of the Chronically Sick and Disabled Persons Act 1970 states that the needs of disabled people should be taken into account when erecting new public buildings 'in so far as it is in the circumstances both practicable and reasonable'. This gives the local authority wide discretionary powers as to what to enforce, and is not applicable to buildings of an older date.

Question 4.3

Several sections of the Chronically Sick and Disabled Persons Act 1970 are relevant here. First the local authority has a duty to inform itself of how many people within its area are disabled, what provisions they are likely to require and the extent of the provisions to be made. Joe may well already be registered as disabled, so the local authority is aware of his needs.

As regards housing under Section 3, local authorities must include the provision they intend making for the disabled in any proposals for new housing. The Act states that the local authority shall 'have regard to the special needs of chronically sick or disabled persons'. However, the local authority has to live within a fixed budget and give priority to some groups of handicapped over others. Joe may not be seen as having a very high priority when it comes to rehousing, but it is well worth him asking as local authorities vary considerably in their interpretation of the Act and the amount of resources they plan to use for the disabled.

Question 4.4

The Occupiers Liability Act 1957 states that the occupier of a property has a duty to provide a safe environment to visitors. Ensuring the maintenance of essential pieces of equipment would be part of this duty. If a visitor suffered harm as a result of the dangerous conditions of the property or failure to ensure the safe working order of equipment, then the occupier could be sued.

The nurse in the patient's home is a visitor and therefore the protection of this legislation applies to her. It is therefore Joe's responsibility to report any malfunction of equipment on loan and to be prepared to forgo his bath in order to safeguard the nurse.

Question 4.5

Yes. As is clear from question 4.4, there is a failure here in the occupier's duty, so Mary is entitled to protect herself. She can, of course, approach the problem from a different angle and offer to give him an all over wash instead.

Question 4.6

1. Report the incident to her senior officer.
2. Complete an accident form.
3. Undergo a medical check to ascertain the severity of the injury and any appropriate treatment.

Question 4.7

The Disabled Persons Employment Act 1944 laid down that employers of 20 or more people should recruit a prescribed percentage of disabled persons (3%). The definition of disabled under this Act is 'a person who, on account of injury, disease or congenital deformity is substantially handicapped in obtaining or keeping employment or in undertaking work on his own account, of a kind which, apart from that injury, disease or deformity would be suited to his age, experience and qualifications'. He must also 'want a job and have a reasonable prospect of obtaining and keeping one'. A voluntary register of these disabled people is kept at local employment offices. However, an employer can apply for a permit to employ non-registered people if there are no registered disabled people or no one who is suitably qualified for the job available.

The Employment and Training Act 1973 calls for provision of courses at Employment Rehabilitation Centres. These are for men and women of any employable age who have been referred by their Disablement Resettlement Officer and who need special help in returning to work. The aim of these centres is for assessment and rehabilitation, rather than retraining. In addition this Act provides for vocational training of disabled people suitable to their age, experience and general qualifications.

The Disabled Persons (Employment) Act amended 1958 legislates for those disabled who cannot be fitted into open employment and introduces the concept of sheltered employment. Such workshops may be run on a local authority, government sponsored or voluntary basis.

Finally, Section 2 of the Chronically Sick and Disabled Persons (Amendment) Act 1976 aims at providing access and facilities for employment for the disabled in offices, shops and factories in order to improve employment opportunities. The provision is 'as far as is reasonable and practicable in the circumstances'.

Question 4.8

The grounds for abortion under the Abortion Act 1967 are:

1. that the continuance of the pregnancy would involve risk to the life of the pregnant woman, or of injury to the physical or mental health of the pregnant woman, or of any existing children of her family, greater than if the pregnancy were terminated;
2. that there is a substantial risk that if the child were born, it would suffer from such physical or mental abnormalities as to be seriously handicapped.

In addition, under the Human Fertilisation and Embryology Act 1990 the following amendments to the 1967 Act are made:

1. a 24 week time limit on the above grounds of risk to the physical or mental health of the pregnant woman or of any existing children of her family;
2. no time limit on the remaining grounds for abortion above;
3. a new ground for abortion of grave permanent injury to the physical or mental health of the pregnant woman, with no time limit.

Question 4.9

Maternity leave and pay entitlements are directly related to length of employment, hours worked and future intentions and act on a sliding scale. If Lara had been working full time, but under 2 years and she intends returning to work, she will be entitled to 18 weeks paid maternity leave with 8 weeks full pay, 10 weeks 1/2 pay with additional lower rate statutory maternity pay (SMP). She would be able to take a further 34 weeks unpaid leave.

Question 4.10

She should ask the local authority social services department which has a duty to keep a register of people who act as child minders on domestic premises for reward. There will also be a register of people who provide day care in non-domestic premises. The social services department has an annual inspection duty and the power to cancel a person's registration if care is seriously inadequate.

Question 4.11

The legal answer may well be no. If Mary gives wrong care she could be liable. However on moral grounds she really has little option. In addition, as a district nurse she will be wearing uniform and a failure to stop and help may be reported by a bystander to her employer. The health authority may criticize Mary for presenting a poor image of the service or even report her to the UKCC.

Question 4.12

In a first aid situation, the care given by a nurse is expected to be of a higher standard than that of an ordinary person. Thus there may be grounds for the patient to sue Mary if she had caused increased damage to his leg. However the law accepts that in such an emergency situation decisions have to be made quickly with inadequate medical backup. Mary could well argue that if she had not taken swift action to maintain the patient's airway, he could have asphyxiated and died, and his damaged leg had to be of secondary importance.

Question 4.13

There may be later suggestions of negligence in that Mary had not carried out the prescribed care. It is therefore important that any reasons for being unable to give care, for example a failure to gain access to the home or a failure by the patient to give consent, are noted.

Mary may also wish to follow this up in some other way. If it is extremely unusual for the woman to be out she may be concerned that the patient is in fact in the home but unable to answer the door. Mary may decide to contact a relative or even the police to follow this up.

Question 4.14

Although Peter is a qualified nurse, he does not yet have the knowledge and experience of his colleagues. Therefore he should:

1. discuss how to assess priorities;
2. ask for information or supervision when faced with new situations;
3. make sure that he always maintains a safe standard of care;

4. always document carefully not just the care he gives, but also the outcomes of that care;
5. undertake extra training in community care, for example study days or a longer course, when offered.

The same principles would apply to anyone working in an area or situation in which he/she is not confident.

Question 4.15

The strongest argument will be to use the law on negligence. She might be able to produce a case, to show not only an increase in the number of patients, but also in the more intense nature of the nurses' work. If this has not been matched by an increase in nursing establishment, she can argue that it is more and more likely that patients will suffer as a result of inadequate care and this could lead to an increase in litigation or complaints by patients to the health authority. She may also put forward the view that the only options open to her would be for the community service to refuse to accept more than a fixed number of patients or for her budget to be increased so that she can employ more nurses!

Question 4.16

1. Ensure that other staff know her whereabouts.
2. Be accompanied by another member of staff.
3. Not to feel that she must be heroic.
4. Ensure that she both locks herself in the car and locks the car when she leaves it.
5. Keep any handbag or equipment hidden.
6. Avoid narrow alleys or ill-lit areas.
7. Keep to the centre of paths.
8. Be prepared to take evasive action if she feels threatened.

Question 4.17

Under both the Health and Safety at Work (etc.) Act 1974 and the law on negligence regarding the provision of a safe system of working, the employer should take reasonable precautions to ensure the safety of nurses at risk. This will include providing:

1. training in preventing and minimizing violence;
2. equipment that will assist in safeguarding staff, for example personal alarms.

However, in the community setting it is difficult for the health authority to take more than fairly minimal precautions and it is therefore particularly important for the nurse to ensure that her superior is informed of any specific risk.

Question 4.18

There are very few circumstances where a nurse can legally refuse to give care to patients. Mary must give her employer a chance to undertake measures to improve her safety. If the employer fails to do so, Mary would be wise to seek advice from her union or professional organization before taking further action, but an outright refusal may lead to disciplinary action.

Question 4.19

The Children Act 1989 has several parts that could be used in order to safeguard a child from abuse. Although it supports the principle of non-intervention in family life unless absolutely necessary, it has a number of powers depending on whether the child is in immediate danger or not. Mary may well want to discuss the problem with her superior before making a decision to contact the social services department.

Question 4.20

Obviously Mary cannot give Carmel care if she is not welcome in the home as the nurse has no legal right of entry. Similarly, if she is asked to leave, she must do so or become a trespasser. Mary could ask Carmel when would be the best time to visit to avoid any unpleasant incidents. If this is impossible, then Mary must document any details of abuse as a reason for her decision not to visit.

RELEVANT STATUTES AND CASES

Abortion Act 1967
Children Act 1989
Chronically Sick and Disabled Persons Act 1970
Chronically Sick and Disabled Persons (Amendment) Act 1976
Disabled Persons Employment Act 1944, amended 1958
Employment and Training Act 1973
Health and Safety at Work (etc.) Act 1974
Human Fertilisation and Embryology Act 1990
Occupiers Liability Act 1957
Re Walker's Application 1987

REFERENCES

Anderson-Ford, D. (1980) *The Social Worker's Law Book*. McGraw-Hill, Maidenhead, Berkshire.

Guthrie, D. (ed.) (1981) *Disability; Legislation and Practice*. Macmillan, London.

Leenders, F. (1990) Children first. *Community Outlook*, July 1990, pp. 4–6.

Rogers, R. and Salvage, J. (1988) *Nurses at Risk*. Heinemann Nursing, Oxford.

Whincup, M. (1982) *Legal Aspects of Medical and Nursing Service*, 3rd edn. Ravenswood, Beckenham, Kent.

Working in an institution 5

Matthew has enjoyed his nurse training so far and now at the end of his first year is particularly looking forward to spending some time in the mental handicap area.

Is there a legal definition of mental handicap?

Question 5.1

Before he started his training Matthew had participated in the care of some mentally handicapped people at a day centre but the setting of his experience over the next 2 weeks is to be hospital based. This hospital is old but Matthew is pleasantly surprised when he walks onto his allocated ward to find that it has a bright and quite homely appearance. The trained nurse in charge, Josie, shows him around, pointing out the day area with easy chairs and television, and the several separate bedroom areas with a maximum of four occupants in each. She explains that there are 20 'patients' in all ranging from 20 to 50 years old, most with quite severe disabilities. Some have been on the ward for a number of years, and several have been admitted within the last 2 months for assessment or to give relatives a rest.

Case Studies in Law and Nursing,
Ann P. Young.
Published in 1992 by
Chapman & Hall, London
ISBN 0 412 44130 6.

Question 5.2   Who is responsible for those with severe mental handicaps when family support cannot be maintained?

Josie asks another nurse, Nadia, to show Matthew what to do. Nadia takes Matthew into one of the bedrooms and tells him to help her get some of the patients up and dressed so that they are ready for breakfast at 8.30 am. She explains that the most severely handicapped stay in bed until after breakfast.

As Nadia and Matthew are dressing one of the women, she suddenly sits on the floor and screams. Nadia continues to dress her while Matthew looks on feeling very uncomfortable. Then Nadia tells Matthew to help her take the woman, still screaming, to the dining area.

Question 5.3   Is Nadia justified in acting in this way?

Several patients remain in bed for breakfast and Matthew is allocated to feed Gloria, a 22 year old who suffered severe brain damage from meningitis as a baby. Before fetching her breakfast he goes to introduce himself to Gloria and ensure that she is sitting up. However, on moving her bed covers he finds that she has wet the bed. Nadia tells him that they will be getting her up after breakfast anyway and not to change the sheets. Matthew wonders how long Gloria has been in this condition but says no more.

Question 5.4   Is there a possibility of negligence in this situation?

Rachel, a health care assistant, brings Gloria's breakfast. Matthew discovers that Gloria is not able to speak much. She seems to enjoy her cereal. When he offers her some scrambled egg she is less pleased and says 'no'. She eventually takes a little off the spoon but immediately spits it out. Matthew decides to leave the egg and try the toast and marmalade, with much greater success. When Rachel returns to clear the dishes, she tells Matthew off for not giving Gloria the egg in spite of Matthew's explanation, and proceeds to force Gloria to eat some of the, by now cold, scrambled egg. Matthew feels very angry at this and goes to Nadia to complain. However Nadia upholds Rachel's action on dietary grounds and tells Matthew he must appreciate the greater knowledge of those who have been working in the area for a long time.

To what extent can a student question the knowledge of his superiors?

Question 5.5

Once breakfast is cleared away, Josie allocates the morning's work to the staff. This appears to be done on a task basis whereas Matthew is used to working in environments where nurse–patient allocation is practised. When Matthew asks about this, Josie explains that their system works quite well as the staff are used to it.

Do nursing staff have a legal duty to regularly update their knowledge and skills?

Question 5.6

> ## Activity 5.1
> Find out what patterns/models are used in organizing nursing care in your health authority.

Matthew persists in his questioning of their approach and Josie, eventually exasperated, tells him he must do as he is told and turns away from him. (Privately she realizes that the staff on this ward are in need of updating and resolves to raise this with her manager.)

Question 5.7   Must a nurse always obey a more senior colleague?

Matthew then turns to Nadia and asks if he can look after Gloria but she is also irritated by Matthew and pretends not to hear him. However, Rachel says that it is all right and that she will be around if he needs any help.

Question 5.8   Is it legally acceptable for the health care assistant to supervise a student nurse?

The next two hours pass quite enjoyably for Matthew. Once Gloria is washed, dressed and in her chair, he finds some games in a cupboard and tries to teach Gloria to do a simple jigsaw puzzle. Before lunch, Josie is to do a drug round and tells Matthew to observe. He prepares to check the drugs with her but she tells him that this is unnecessary in this hospital. Matthew asks why.

Is it legal for one nurse to check drugs on her own?   *Question 5.9*

Activity 5.2
Read the UKCC leaflet on *Administration of Medicines*, Section 4(g) and (h).

In spite of Josie's explanation, Matthew is quite sure that this is contrary to the health authority's drug policy.

Should Matthew report the nurse?   *Question 5.10*

After this incident, Matthew decides to 'keep his head down' as he realizes he is upsetting the staff. That afternoon he is asked to take one of the more able patients, Tim, for a walk in the hospital grounds. Tim seems very keen to go out and once in the garden asks if they can go to the shop as he has some money to spend. Matthew suggests Tim show him the whereabouts of this shop and they soon find themselves outside the hospital grounds. The shop, a general store, is a few minutes walk along the road. Once there Tim picks out a number of items, after a lot of discussion with Matthew. However, when Tim comes to pay for them he does not have enough money and begins to get very distressed at having to give some of the items back. Matthew feels awkward and offers to pay the difference. Tim quickly forgets his distress and is very pleased with his purchases.

Should Matthew have put his own money towards Tim's purchases?   *Question 5.11*

Once back on the ward, Tim shows off his shopping to the others. Nadia asks him where he got the money to pay for these things but at that Tim insists he has plenty of money and goes to his bedroom to put his things away. Nadia is very concerned and questions Matthew about what happened as she knows that Tim had spent all of his weekly allowance and the next amount is not due for several days.

Activity 5.3
Find out what money is due to longstay patients in hospital and how this is given to them in your organization.

Nadia suspects that Tim may have taken the money from another patient.

Question 5.12   What should the nurse do in these circumstances?

Nadia is also critical of Matthews's action in allowing Tim to leave the hospital as the instruction was for Tim to walk in the hospital grounds only. However, Matthew argues that he was given inadequate information to justify restraining Tim from leaving the hospital.

What information could have been given to Matthew to help him act appropriately when Tim expressed a wish to go shopping?   *Question 5.13*

Matthew has a further nine days on that ward and finds it difficult to fit in and avoid being critical of some of the things he sees. At the end of this time, Josie has to write a report on Matthew's progress. This report states that Matthew's performance has been unsatisfactory on a number of counts. His relationships with the staff have been poor, he is often inconsiderate of others, refuses to accept criticism and is very self-opinionated. When the report is given to him, Matthew is very angry and threatens to take Josie to court for libel.

What is libel?   *Question 5.14*

Would Matthew have any chance of successfully suing for libel in these circumstances?   *Question 5.15*

Once his tutor in the School of Nursing has received the report, she calls a meeting with Matthew to review his progress. He is told he may bring a friend or union representative with him. As Matthew has joined a union, he brings a shop steward with him.

Question 5.16   Why is it advisable, even as a student, to join a union or professional body?

Activity 5.4

Find out what unions or professional bodies a nurse can join and what they offer.

During the meeting, Matthew is asked to state his side of the story. The senior tutor is concerned by some of the facts disclosed and asks why Matthew had not contacted her earlier about these difficulties. He answers that he had not seen the point of doing so.

Question 5.17   Who is responsible for student nurses when they are undertaking clinical experience?

Activity 5.5

Find out what criteria your training establishment uses to accept a clinical area as being suitable for nurse training.

While the senior tutor appreciates a number of Matthew's difficulties, she feels that he has not helped the situation by his manner as on previous occasions staff have commented on this as being rather arrogant. She suggests that in the future Matthew asks for help and support at an early stage if he encounters difficulties.

After the meeting Matthew's union representative suggests that no further action is necessary but points out that if a number of students had found similar difficulties in their training, they might have been able to use the health authority's grievance policy.

Activity 5.6

Find out how to make a grievance in line with your local policy and in what situations a student nurse could use this mechanism.

Shortly after this experience, the tutor for mental handicap training speaks to Matthew about his placement. They discuss some of the problems of caring for the mentally handicapped within an institutional setting and she suggests that Matthew keep an open mind until he has had the opportunity to observe other ways of caring for these 'clients' in a community setting.

What government reports advocated a move from institutionalized to community care for people with mental handicaps?

Question 5.18

ANSWERS

Question 5.1

A number of Acts refer to the handicapped in fairly general terms, for example the National Assistance Act 1948, the Public Health Act 1936, amended 1968, and the Chronically Sick and Disabled Persons Act 1970. However these do not give any kind of precise definition of mental handicap. The Mental Health Act 1983 defines two categories, mental impairment and severe mental impairment.

Severe mental impairment means a state of arrested or incomplete development of mind which includes severe impairment of intelligence and social functioning and is associated with abnormally aggressive or seriously irresponsible conduct. Mental impairment means a state of arrested or incomplete development of mind (not amounting to severe mental impairment) which includes significant impairment of intelligence and social functioning and is associated with abnormally aggressive or seriously irresponsible conduct.

The majority of those with a mental handicap are outside these definitions. The significance of this is that only those with aggressive or seriously irresponsible behaviour can be admitted compulsorily to hospital.

Question 5.2

The local authority has a duty to provide services and care to disabled people. The health service has a responsibility to assess and treat those admitted under the Mental Health Act 1983 (see definitions above). However, prior to the 1983 Act, the Mental Health Act 1959 had a definition of subnormality that was much broader and meant that mentally handicapped people were more likely to be admitted to hospital. It is relatively recently that the move to caring for the mentally handicapped in the community has been supported by Parliament and an increase in appropriate Community Services.

Question 5.3

To some extent Nadia is legally justified in assuming the patient's consent to being dressed as she initially cooperated and even when she started screaming she did not actively refuse to be dressed. Whether Nadia can justify her actions on ethical and practical grounds would depend on whether this situation had arisen previously and if so what alternative approaches had been employed to gain the patient's active cooperation.

Question 5.4

The staff owe Gloria a duty of care to keep her clean and dry, and in this situation there may well be a failure in that duty. However, for negligence there must be resultant harm, the most likely being excoriation or breakdown of the skin. How quickly this happened would depend on a number of factors as well as how long the patient had been left in a wet bed, so this part of negligence might be difficult to prove.

Question 5.5

On the one hand, it is important for a student to question as that is a way to learn. However, without a broad knowledge base it is difficult for a student to appreciate all the reasons why certain decisions are made. Choosing between two less than ideal solutions is also problematic. In Gloria's situation there is a potential legal difficulty of choosing between assault and battery in forcing her to eat or negligence in failing to give her an adequate diet. As in question 5.3, the real issue may be that there are other practical approaches that also gain the patient's cooperation and the thoughtful student may be able to suggest a satisfactory alternative.

Question 5.6

Yes, when a change in nursing care has been widely documented and evaluated as being of benefit to the patient there is an expectation in law that a nurse will have updated herself and have implemented change accordingly. However, in this particular situation it may be extremely difficult to pin-point resultant harm for failing to implement a different model of care as there are so many other variables affecting the progress that patients make.

Question 5.7

A nurse must have a very good reason for refusing to obey a senior colleague otherwise she is likely to be disciplined or even dismissed. The only sound reasons are:

1. in order to avoid participating in a criminal or negligent act;
2. if she has expressed an objection under the Abortion Act 1967;
3. to avoid putting herself into a situation of marked danger particularly when her employer has made no attempt to remedy or reduce this or is expecting the employee to act unreasonably.

Question 5.8

No. The National Boards require that a student is supervised by a registered nurse although there is no reason why the student and health care assistant should not work together if both are competent in what they are doing. However the registered nurse does need to know what tasks are being undertaken by the student as she could well be negligent in supervision if harm resulted from a student's incompetence.

Question 5.9

There is no statute that legislates on how drugs must be checked prior to administration. It is therefore quite legal for only one nurse to check drugs. Legislation applies to the ordering, storage, prescription and recording of drugs.

Question 5.10

There is no legal requirement to report another person's wrongdoing. Professionally the UKCC Code of Professional Conduct states that the nurse should 'act always in such a way as to promote and safeguard the wellbeing and interest of patient/clients' and therefore the nurse has a duty to protect her patients from poor practice. In Matthew's situation he could try to assess the risks to the patients himself but would be better advised to take advice from someone more experienced.

Question 5.11

In retrospect Matthew would have been wiser to have checked how much money the patient had before going into the shop. However, in the circumstances as long as the amount of money was small Matthew could have lent the patient some of his own money on the understanding that this was reimbursed. For this, Matthew would need a receipt from the shop which he could have shown the ward staff.

Question 5.12

She must inform the nurse in charge. Together they could question Tim as well as checking his property and his records but this will not necessarily be helpful in pin-pointing whether Tim took any money. The security officer (if there is one) could also be contacted. It is unlikely that the police would be called in at this point. Even if evidence was found against Tim, the police would be unwilling to press charges. For there to be a conviction for theft there must be the dishonest intention to permanently deprive another of his goods. This intention may be difficult to prove with someone like Tim whose mental age is low. A result of this concern should be a review of how patients' money is controlled and what security measures are available.

Question 5.13

1. Whether Tim was used to going outside the hospital grounds.
2. Why on this occasion Tim was to stay within the hospital grounds.
3. What techniques to use to persuade Tim against or distract him from leaving the hospital.
4. How to get help or advice if needed.

The failure of the trained staff to ensure that such information was given to Matthew could potentially have been negligent.

Question 5.14

Libel is a form of defamation and is a statement made in permanent form, usually writing, that exposes a person to hatred, ridicule or contempt or causes him to be shunned or avoided by 'right-thinking' members of society.

Question 5.15

He is unlikely to be successful if the following conditions apply:

1. The statements are true and Josie can support their accuracy by giving specific examples of Matthew's behaviour.
2. The report is only shown to Matthew and Matthew's tutor in which case the report is the subject of privilege as it has been written and divulged only in the course of duty.

Question 5.16

1. For protection in case legal action is taken against the nurse.
2. For advice and to act for the nurse if she wishes to take legal action herself on some matter relating to her employment or training.
3. To ensure that the nurse's interests and rights are safeguarded in any disciplinary or dismissal situations.
4. To provide assistance with settling grievances.
5. For a vote on negotiating bodies where decision on pay and conditions are made.

Question 5.17

The educational establishment has overall responsibility for the student throughout her course. Although the clinical nurses have to be responsible for the supervision, teaching and assessment of learners in their area, any decisions concerning a student's progress or the suitability or otherwise of a clinical area for training must be made by the school or college.

Question 5.18

Community Care: an agenda for action. Report to the Secretary of State for Social Services (1988) by Sir Roy Griffiths is the most recent and culminated in The Community Care Act 1990. The Cumberledge Report, *Neighbourhood Nursing – A Focus for Care* (1988) was also influential, following on the *Jay Report* (1979), the *Short Report* (1985) and the DHSS consultative document *Care in the Community* (1981).

RELEVANT STATUTES AND CASES

Abortion Act 1967
Chronically Sick and Disabled Persons Act 1970
Mental Health Act 1959

Mental Health Act 1983
Misuse of Drugs Act 1971
National Assistance Act 1948
National Health Service and Community Care Act 1990
Public Health Act 1936, amended 1968
Theft Act 1968
Clarke *v.* MacLennan 1983
Hunter *v.* Hanley 1955

REFERENCES

Brazier, M. (1987) *Medicine, Patients and the Law*. Penguin, Harmondsworth, Middlesex.

Medical Defence Union (1986) *Consent to Treatment*. Medical Defence Union, London.

Parish, A. (ed.) (1987) *Mental Handicap*. Macmillan, London.

Taylor, J. (1986) *Mental Handicap: Partnership in the Community?* Office of Health Economics, London.

United Kingdom Central Council (1984) *Code of Professional Conduct*, 2nd edn. UKCC, London.

United Kingdom Central Council (1986) *Administration of Medicines, a UKCC Advisory Paper*. UKCC, London.

Standards of care   6

Until 4 weeks ago, 7-year-old Rudie was a lively child, active and full of energy. His sudden lethargy and inability to shake off a cold he has caught, lead his mother to take him to the general practitioner, who takes blood for tests.

Should a doctor inform a patient of why blood is being taken?

Question 6.1

The results of these tests are abnormal and the GP asks for an urgent appointment for Rudie with the hospital consultant. Two weeks later Rudie and his parents, Priscilla and George, are waiting in the Out-Patient Department. At the nearby reception desk, the receptionist and a nurse are talking about another patient in loud voices. George and Priscilla cannot help overhearing a number of details concerning this patient's illness and personal life.

Are the receptionist and nurse acting illegally in this situation?

Question 6.2

Activity 6.1
Read the UKCC leaflet on *Confidentiality*, pp. 8–9.

Case Studies in Law and Nursing,
Ann P. Young.
Published in 1992 by
Chapman & Hall, London
ISBN 0 412 44130 6.

When the family are seen by the consultant, he explains that there are some abnormalities in Rudie's blood but until further tests are carried out, it will not be possible to know what is wrong. He says that he would like to admit Rudie to the children's ward in a week's time in order that more extensive tests can be carried out. Rudie's parents are understandably worried but accept the necessity for this action.

On the way out, they ask the nurse at the reception desk what they will need to do about Rudie's admission. She explains that details will be sent to them and in the meantime gives Rudie a booklet about coming into hospital. She tells Priscilla and George to try not to worry as leukaemia is often treatable in children. They are so shocked at this that they say no more and quickly leave the department. However, once home, George telephones the hospital and speaks to the consultant who explains that leukaemia is one potential diagnosis but that there are other possibilities.

Question 6.3   Is it permissible for a nurse to tell the patient or relatives a medical diagnosis?

Priscilla decides to write to the hospital about the nurse concerned, complaining both about the way she told them of Rudie's possible diagnosis and the manner in which she was breaching confidentiality earlier in their visit.

Question 6.4   What might be the outcome of these complaints for this nurse?

Activity 6.2

Find out from the most recent UKCC reports available to you, the reasons for nurses having to appear before the professional conduct committee.

A week later, Rudie, accompanied by his mother, enters Cameron Ward. Staff nurse Sally Davies explains what will be happening and it is not long before the doctor arrives to take more blood samples. After this Rudie soon becomes engrossed in helping another child build a model fire engine and Priscilla feels happy to leave him with the play leader. On the way out of the ward, she notices that the door handle is unusually high and that the door automatically closes behind her.

Why are these safety features important in a paediatric ward?

Question 6.5

Activity 6.3

See how many safety features you can find in your nearest children's ward, creche or play group.

After a number of investigations have been completed, the consultant interviews George and Priscilla in a side room. He breaks the news that Rudie does indeed have leukaemia. However, it has been diagnosed at a fairly early stage and there is a good chance that Rudie can be cured. George and Priscilla stay there alone for ten minutes to compose themselves before returning to Rudie, but even so Rudie senses that something has happened and asks if the doctor knows what is wrong with him. His parents hug him and tell him that he is going to be all right. They then leave to fetch some items from home so that they can be resident in the hospital during Rudie's stay. Not long after, Sally finds him huddled in his bed crying. Between sobs, he tells her he must be very ill because nobody will tell him what is wrong.

Question 6.6   Does a child have a right to be given information about his illness and treatment?

Question 6.7   What role can the nurse play in such a situation?

A decision is made to treat Rudie's leukaemia with cytotoxic drugs and the consent of his parents is sought.

Question 6.8   At what age is a child considered to be capable of giving a valid consent for himself?

Rudie's parents are initially hesitant in giving their consent as the treatment seems to them to be so traumatic as well as carrying a number of risks. However, after further explanation and discussion they agree to the treatment.

Question 6.9   If parents withhold their consent, can they be overruled?

At this point the consultant spends some time with Rudie explaining what is wrong with him and the treatment he is going to have. Rudie says he will work very hard to get better and do everything that the doctors and nurses want. It is decided to use a new drug regime. Initial research into this has shown promising results but it is still an experimental approach rather than a well-established regime.

What legal constraints are there to carrying out medical research or experimental treatments?

Question 6.10

Activity 6.4
Drug trials are the most common type of medical research involving the nurse. Find out what procedures are followed in your health authority in order to safeguard the patients involved.

Intensive treatment intravenously via a Hickman line takes place over the next two weeks. Rudie becomes very weak and tired which Priscilla finds distressing although she has been warned of this. The nurses encourage her to help care for Rudie so she washes him each day and helps to keep his mouth as fresh as possible although it rapidly becomes sore as a side effect of the drugs. Priscilla worries that she may dislodge the intravenous lines into Rudie or damage his mouth but the nurses reassure her that they will help her and show her how to care for him safely.

Question 6.11   Is it legally acceptable for relatives to participate in the care of a patient?

The nurses also encourage Priscilla to help Rudie take adequate nourishment. One evening she prepares a hot drink for him in the ward kitchen. As she uses the hot water geyser, she splashes boiling water on her hand which she quickly rinses under the cold water tap. However a nurse also present in the kitchen insists on reporting the incident to the nurse in charge who completes an accident form.

Question 6.12   What legal responsibilities do the ward staff have towards accidental injuries to visitors?

Several days into the treatment, Priscilla is surprised to see the nurses coming on duty in their ordinary clothes although they put colourful aprons on when undertaking some tasks. She asks them what is going on and is told they are running a trial in the paediatric ward on the benefits or hazards of wearing ordinary clothes rather than uniforms. The experiment is to last one month and will be carefully evaluated.

What legal precautions must be taken when considering setting up an experiment affecting nursing care?

Question 6.13

Assuming a reasonably successful outcome to this experiment, how could the ward nurses go about implementing a change in the uniform policy?

Question 6.14

Once Rudie's intensive treatment is completed, the doctors suggest he goes home to continue his ongoing treatment there with the community nurse in attendance. Although he is still a very sick child, the thought of going home pleases Rudie so his parents and the hospital staff make the necessary arrangements.

The community paediatric liaison nurse, Tessa, calls only two hours after they arrive home and explains what her role will be over the coming weeks. She will advise Priscilla and George on how to nurse Rudie with particular attention to his oral hygiene and diet. In addition she will be injecting his drugs via his Hickman line.

Question 6.15   On what basis can the nurse take on these responsibilities?

As the days go by, Rudie's mouth gets sorer and develops white patches. Tessa explains that it has become infected and that he will have to suck some special lozenges. Rudie is feeling very irritable and blames his mother as she has been cleaning his mouth for him; Priscilla blames the hospital nurse for not showing her how to do this properly.

Question 6.16   Is there any negligence in this situation?

When Tessa has a day off, another nurse covers for her. Priscilla is surprised and confused when this nurse gives some totally contrary advice on Rudie's diet to that given by Tessa. Priscilla decides to ignore this advice and check with Tessa when she returns as to which diet is best.

Question 6.17   What are the legal implications of giving wrong advice to a patient?

On Tessa's return, she reassures Priscilla by giving her a booklet about diet for patients having cytotoxic drugs.

Rudie's condition gradually improves as his drug dosage is reduced and physically he becomes stronger although he is still very under-weight. His blood tests are also encouraging although treatment, including some as an inpatient, will have to continue for several years. Priscilla and George are so relieved that Rudie has been given a chance of cure and so grateful to Tessa for her support and care that they decide to give her a cheque for £20.00 and a silver necklace.

How should Tessa respond to these gifts?

Question 6.18

> *Activity 6.5*
> Read the UKCC's Code of Professional Conduct and identify which sections have been relevant to this case sutdy.

ANSWERS

Question 6.1

Yes. The patient should give consent not just to the taking of blood but to the tests to be performed on that sample. This issue has become of par-ticular significance in the anonymous testing of blood for HIV infection. However, it still seems to be common practice for staff taking blood samples to assume consent unless the patient specifically asks for further information.

Question 6.2

The nurse and receptionist have a clear duty to maintain confidentiality, but there is no specific law to prevent such a breach or to ensure that there is a legal outcome. The law on defamation can occasionally be used, but the nature of the confidential information disclosed is rarely defamatory in nature. In Scotland, if a breach of confidentiality leads to harm, then the nurse may possibly be liable for damages.

Question 6.3

Legally it is the duty of the doctor to give information on a patient's diagnosis. He is legally in charge of the patient and also has ownership of any medical knowledge relating to the patient. There are, of course, a number of occasions when the situation may not be as clear-cut as suggested by the legal position, for example when a patient or relative wishes to be given confirmation of what he suspects or asks for additional information. However, there is no doubt that the nurse acted wrongly both on legal and ethical grounds in leaking the possible diagnosis of leukaemia in such inappropriate and unsolicited circumstances.

Question 6.4

There are several possible outcomes:

1. The nurse is likely to be disciplined by her manager for acting unprofessionally on both counts.
2. She may also be found to be in breach of her contract if this specifically includes a clause requiring that confidentiality be maintained. This would also lead to disciplinary action but could even result in dismissal.
3. The employer may decide to report the nurse to the UKCC. If it is decided that the allegations of misconduct must be taken further, the case is forwarded to the professional conduct committee of the UKCC. This committee has to prove whether or not the incidents occurred and, if so, whether they constitute professional misconduct. If they do, the nurse may have her name removed from the Register, have no action taken apart from being referred to the Code of Professional Conduct or judgement may be postponed to give time for certain criteria to be met. A fourth option is to refer the nurse to the health committee if the professional conduct committee suspect her actions have been influenced by her state of health.

Question 6.5

The duty of the hospital authority to prevent harm occurring to patients is increased when those patients are less able to take responsibility themselves. This is apparent with young children who could suffer damage if they left the ward unsupervised. For example, a child falling downstairs could demonstrate negligence if no precautions were taken to prevent this happening.

Question 6.6

The answer to this depends on the understanding of the child. There is no legal reason for not giving the child information. Staff and parents often underestimate the ability of the child to accept and come to terms with unpleasant facts. However, the rights of any patient to demand that information is given are dependent on the doctor's opinion as to whether such information will cause severe mental harm. On the other hand, to mislead the patient by giving inadequate information may be negligence if harm resulted.

Question 6.7

As was seen in question 6.3, the nurse is legally constrained in what she can tell the patient. However she can play an important role by ensuring that the doctor is told of Rudie's distress at not knowing what is wrong, by going over with the patient what has happened so far and what might be happening in the future, by giving further explanation of facts already given but not properly understood and by reassuring Rudie that she will help as far as she possibly can in giving him information when she is able to.

Question 6.8

This is normally considered to be 16 years old in spite of the age of majority being 18 years. Parents cannot veto any treatment that the 16 or 17 year old is willing to accept. However, in an emergency if there is inadequate time to contact the parents or guardian the child's consent is considered sufficient if he is able to understand what is proposed.

Question 6.9

In certain circumstances the refusal of parents or guardian can be overruled. Parents have responsibilities for their children and one of these duties is to provide the necessary medical aid. Thus if certain treatment is urgently needed to save life or to prevent some marked disability that would seriously affect the child's future, the doctor or nurse can proceed without the parent's consent. In some situations a special court order can be obtained from the duty magistrate. The local authority then gives consent in place of the parents. The child could also be made a ward of court.

Question 6.10

Although there are a number of codes that give guidance on the principles to be followed when carrying out experiments on patients (the Nuremberg Code 1948 and the Declaration of Helsinki 1975), these do not have legal status. The laws relating to negligence and consent have to be used.

As with gaining consent for other treatments, the principle of the more urgent the need for treatment, the less the requirement to give detailed information would apply. Most experimental treatments fall into the remit of not being immediately necessary so the doctor has a greater duty to give information. However, the efficacy of some experiments may possibly be reduced by giving a great deal of information so that the doctor faces conflicting needs. As it is the doctor who makes the decision as to how much information to give, this seems to give the patient limited legal rights.

The law assumes that the doctor will carry out treatment with reasonable skill and knowledge. This will also apply where new or little tried treatments are to be used and therefore there will be negligence if he fails to take reasonable care in the circumstances.

Question 6.11

This situation arises quite frequently in many areas of nursing but is particularly relevant in the paediatric area. As long as the relative voluntarily takes on this care with the approval of the nursing staff and the care given is that normally undertaken by a relative in the home, then it is likely that the hospital will legally accept this participation. Where the care given requires a nursing skill that has to be particularly learnt by the relative, then additional constraints must apply and the delegation of such care to a relative must only be done with the permission of senior management and with stringent precautions, including proper training.

Question 6.12

Under the Occupiers Liability Act 1957, the hospital has a duty to protect visitors from harm due to negligence on the part of its staff. Therefore if a visitor does sustain an injury this must be reported. In Priscilla's situation, she had been encouraged to participate in Rudie's needs and allowed to use the kitchen. If it was known that the geyser was faulty, she should have been warned.

Question 6.13

As with medical experimentation, the nurses must avoid negligence and should therefore consider what risks there might be to the patients in wearing ordinary clothes rather than uniform. In addition, nurses are required contractually to abide by hospital policies, including the uniform policy. Any deviation from this must be agreed by senior management to avoid incurring disciplinary action.

Question 6.14

As hospital policies are binding on the employees of the health authority, certain formal channels must be used in order to change those policies. The nurses involved in the experiment in the children's ward would need to present their findings and request to change the uniform policy to senior management. The usual route would then be for a draft amendment to the policy to be drawn up and circulated to interested parties. These will include managers and staff in the paediatric unit as well as union representatives. Once comments are received an amended policy can be presented to the senior management group for approval. Once approved, the new policy will be circulated and implemented.

Question 6.15

The paediatric liaison nurse's role includes components which are not normally part of general or, to any marked extent, paediatric nurse training. The knowledge of specific paediatric dietary requirements and the expertise for giving drugs via a Hickman line are beyond the skills expected of most registered nurses.

For a nurse to take on these extra duties certain requirements must apply:

1. The profession and the employer must have accepted the suitability of a nurse taking on these tasks.
2. The nurse must have been specifically and adequately trained.
3. The training must have been accepted as satisfactory by the employer.
4. The doctor must be satisfied that the nurse is competent to give drugs via the Hickman line.
5. The nurse must accept the delegation of these duties to her and only undertake them when she feels competent to do so.

Question 6.16

The only possible negligence could be if the hospital nurse had shown Priscilla a faulty technique, but as the mouth infection has occurred several weeks after Priscilla first started cleaning Rudie's mouth, negligence is extremely unlikely. The most likely reason for Rudie's mouth infection is as a side effect of the cytotoxic drugs which reduce the body's normal resistance to infection. Patients (and their relatives) have to accept that some harm is an unavoidable risk of treatment.

Question 6.17

Wrong advice can lead to negligence if harm results to a patient (or relative) following this faulty information. It may sometimes be difficult to prove resultant harm as the harm may not become apparent for some time and other factors may also be at work.

Question 6.18

Tessa should refuse gifts of any marked monetary value and she should certainly refuse to accept money. The reason for this is that later, the parents may regret their generosity and claim that they were put under pressure to give the nurse gifts. The nurse may then face accusations of corruption.

However Tessa should be understanding of the motives that have prompted the gifts and grateful to Priscilla and George for their appreciation. If the necklace is not an expensive one, she may feel able to receive this, but should in any event inform her manager of what has occurred and ensure that she abides by any local policies regarding the acceptance of gifts.

RELEVANT STATUTES AND CASES

Children Act 1989
Family Law Reform Act 1969
Nurses, Midwives and Health Visitors Act 1979
Occupiers Liability Act 1957
Prevention of Corruption Act 1906 and 1916
Wilsher *v.* Essex AHA 1986–1988

REFERENCES

Department of Health (1989) *An Introduction to the Children Act 1989.* HMSO, London.
Department of Health and Social Security (1977) *The Extending Role of the Clinical Nurse – Legal Implications and Training Requirements,* HC(77)22. DHSS, London.
Dimond, B. (1990) Parental acts and omissions, *Paediatric Nursing,* Feb. 1990, pp. 23–4.
Mason, J.K. and McCall Smith, R.A. (1987) *Law and Medical Ethics,* 2nd edn. Butterworth, London.
Tingle, J.H. (1989) Extending capability. *Nursing Standard,* **4** (6), 32.
United Kingdom Central Council (1984) *Code of Professional Conduct,* 2nd edn. UKCC, London.
United Kingdom Central Council (1987) *Confidentiality, a UKCC Advisory Paper.* UKCC, London.
Young, A.P. (1989) *Legal Problems in Nursing Practice,* 2nd edn. Harper and Row, London.
Young, A.P. (1991) *Law and Professional Conduct in Nursing.* Scutari Press, London.

PART TWO
Branch Programmes – Level 2

Adult nursing   7

Alan was diagnosed several years ago as suffering from AIDS. He had been maintained in reasonable health for some time with the use of prophylactic drugs but over the last six months his condition has deteriorated. His partner, Ray, has been caring for him at home for as long as possible but Alan now needs facilities and equipment that can only be provided in hospital. Although the hospital has an AIDS unit, there are no beds available there at present so Alan has to be admitted to a general medical ward and placed in a side room. He is very weak and emaciated and seems withdrawn. His skin is in a poor state and his breathing sounds laboured.

On the day of Alan's admission there are three trained nurses on duty along with one auxiliary nurse and two students. The staff nurse in charge is approached by the other nurses for advice on nursing Alan. They express the opinion that Alan should not have been admitted to their ward as they have neither the knowledge nor experience of nursing patients with AIDS. One staff nurse, Zita, says that she will not care for him as the risk of having the HIV infection passed to her is too great. One of the students, Paul, says that this is a load of rubbish. He has a number of friends who are homosexuals and therefore at higher risk of carrying the HIV virus and there are no risks of catching AIDS from them by normal social contact. After some heated discussion, including insinuations made that if Paul is a practising homosexual he should not be nursing, the staff nurse in charge bleeps the control of infection nursing officer for help.

Read the material below before answering questions 7.1–7.4. You may also find of use the following answers:

Chapter 2 Nos. 8 and 14
Chapter 4 Nos. 17 and 18
Chapter 5 No. 8
Chapter 6 Nos. 2 and 4

(A) PUBLIC HEALTH ACT (INFECTIOUS DISEASE) REGULATIONS 1985

Case Studies in Law and Nursing, Ann P. Young. Published in 1992 by Chapman & Hall, London ISBN 0 412 44130 6.

1. Gives to local authorities the power to apply to a Justice of the Peace for the removal of an AIDS sufferer to hospital to be detained there.
2. Gives to the JP the power to make an order for a person believed to be

suffering from AIDS to be medically examined. There are also powers in relation to the disposal of the body of an AIDS sufferer.

(B) AIDS CONTROL ACT 1987

This Act requires District Health Authorities to report to the Regional Health Authorities (or Welsh Office) and for the regional authorities to report to the Secretary of State, giving information set out in the schedule and other such relevant information as the Secretary of State may direct. The schedule includes the following:

1. the number of persons known to be persons with AIDS and the timing of the diagnosis;
2. the particulars of facilities and services provided by each authority;
3. the numbers of persons employed by the authority in providing such facilities;
4. future provision over the next 12 months.

It also requires details of the action taken to educate members of the public in relation to AIDS and HIV, to provide training for testing for AIDS, and for the treatment, counselling and care of persons with AIDS or infected with HIV.

A subsequent statutory instrument has extended the information required to include HIV positive persons (Aids (Control) (Contents of Reports Order) 1988 Section 117).

(C) ABORTION ACT 1967

Section 4: No person shall be under any duty, whether by contract or by any statutory or other legal requirement, to participate in any treatment authorized by this Act to which he has a conscientious objection. Provided that in any legal proceedings the burden of proof of conscientious objection shall rest on the person claiming to rely on it.

Nothing in the above section shall effect any duty to participate in treatment which is necessary to save the life or to prevent grave permanent injury to the physical or mental health of a pregnant woman.

(D) SACKED ECT NURSE LOSES APPEAL

Martin Vousden

A psychiatric nurse who was dismissed for refusing to participate in electro-convulsive therapy (ECT) lost his appeal at an employment tribunal last week.

Derek Owen, a former staff nurse at Walsgrave Hospital, Coventry, was appealing against the findings of an industrial tribunal held in Birmingham which decided that he had disobeyed a lawful and reasonable instruction to help give ECT treatment.

The findings of the industrial tribunal were upheld because Mr Owen's contract stated that participation in ECT might be part of his work.

In his judgement, Mr Justice Popplewell said that no employee was required to do something that was dangerous to a third party but what Mr Owen was asked to do conflicted with his perception of what was in the patient's best interests.

This was a decision for the medical staff said Justice Popplewell, and was not sufficient reason for Mr Owen to refuse to administer ECT.

After the hearing Mr Owen said 'This decision abolishes all the claims of nurses right across the country, to use any clinical judgement whatever. It is an abysmal judgement which makes it difficult for nurses to function as members of a multidisciplinary team.

For me, the crucial thing is to await the response of the professional organisations. I think that one or other of them should be taking up this issue. If they don't, I'm not sure that I have the personal resources to follow it through.'

Martin Brown, assistant nurse adviser to the RCN Society of Psychiatric Nursing, said: 'We are astonished by the implications of the decision taken by the court, which seems to suggest that nurses are not responsible for their own practice.'

He said the society would be eager to study the transcript of the hearing and would be discussing the issue at the next society meeting in December.

Mr Owen had based his argument in court on the UKCC Code of Professional Conduct. His barrister had argued that, according to the code, a nurse should not do anything which was not in the patient's best interests.

It should, therefore, be a matter of public policy, he said, not to instruct nurses to do anything which they believed could be harmful to patients.

Keith Hickson, national officer for COHSE, commented: 'This case highlights a matter of growing concern. Section six of the UKCC code of professional conduct sows potential seeds of conflict between the nurse and doctors or hospital managers.

Section six gives an implied responsibility to nurses to express their views when they have genuine and legitimate grounds for concern about proposed treatment. But they have no real framework in which they can express that concern.

The law courts are not a satisfactory way of resolving ethical problems.'

Reg Pyne, the UKCC's director for professional conduct, said: 'This is potentially a significant issue.'

Bill Bingley, legal director with the National Association for Mental Health, told NM: 'We feel there is a need for some provision for nurses not to be forced to participate in treatments about which they have strong moral or ethical reservations.'

Nursing Mirror (14.11.84)

(E) UKCC CODE OF PROFESSIONAL CONDUCT (1984) (RELEVANT SECTIONS)

Each registered nurse, midwife and health visitor shall act, at all times, in such a manner as to justify public trust and confidence, to uphold and enhance the good standing and reputation of the profession, to serve the interests of society, and above all to safeguard the interests of individual patients and clients.

Each registered nurse, midwife and health visitor is accountable for his or her practice, and, in the exercise of professional accountability shall:

1. Act always in such a way as to promote and safeguard the well-being and interests of patients/clients.
2. Ensure that no action or omission on his/her part or within his/her sphere of influence is detrimental to the condition or safety of patients/clients.
3. Take every reasonable opportunity to maintain and improve professional knowledge and competence.
10. Have regard to the environment of care and its physical, psychological and social effects on patients/clients, and also to the adequacy of resources, and make known to appropriate persons or authorities any circumstances which could place patients/clients in jeopardy or which militate against safe standards of practice.

UKCC (1984)

(F) HEALTH AND SAFETY AT WORK (ETC.) ACT 1974

Section 2

General duties of employers to their employees

1. It shall be the duty of every employer to ensure, so far as it is reasonably practicable, the health, safety and welfare at work of all his employees.
2. Without prejudice to the generality of an employer's duty under the preceding subsection, the matters to which that duty extends include in particular:
   (a) the provision and maintenance of plant and systems of work that are, so far as is reasonably practical, safe and without risks to health;
   (b) arrangements for ensuring, so far as is reasonably practicable, safety and absence of risks to health in connection with the use, handling, storage and transport of articles and substances;
   (c) the provision of such information, instruction, training and supervision as is necessary to ensure, so far as is reasonably practicable, the health and safety at work of his employee;
   (d) so far as is reasonably practicable as regards any place of work under the employer's control, the maintenance of it in a condition that is safe and without risks to health and the provision and maintenance of means of access to and egress from it that are safe and without such risks;
   (e) the provision and maintenance of a working environment for his employees that is so far as is reasonably practicable, safe, without risks to health and adequate as regards facilities and arrangements for their welfare at work.

3. Except in such cases as may be prescribed, it shall be the duty of every employer to prepare and as often as may be appropriate revise a written statement of his general policy with respect to the health and safety at work of his employees and the organization and arrangements for the time being in force for carrying out that policy and to bring the statement and any revision of it to the notice of all his employees.

4. Regulations made by the Secretary of State may provide for the appointment in prescribed cases by recognized trade unions (within the meaning of the regulations) of safety representatives from amongst the employees, and those representatives shall represent the employees in consultations with the employers under subsection (6) below and shall have such other functions as may be prescribed.

5. Repealed.

6. It shall be the duty of every employer to consult any such representatives with a view to the making and maintenance of arrangements which will enable him and his employees to cooperate effectively in promoting and developing measures to ensure the health and safety at work of the employees, and in checking the effectiveness of such measures.

7. In such cases as may be prescribed it shall be the duty of every employer, if requested to do so by the safety representatives mentioned in subsections (4) and (5) above, to establish, in accordance with regulations made by the Secretary of State, a safety committee having the function of keeping under review the measures taken to ensure the health and safety at work of his employees and such other functions as may be prescribed.

Section 7

It shall be the duty of every employee while at work:
   (a) to take reasonable care for the health and safety of himself and of others who may be affected by his acts or omissions at work;
   (b) as regards any duty or requirement imposed on his employer or other person by or under any of the relevant statutory provisions to cooperate with him in so far as is necessary to enable that duty or requirement to be performed or complied with.

(G) NATIONAL HEALTH SERVICE (AMENDMENT) ACT 1986

Section 1 of the Act provides for the application of food legislation to health authorities and health service premises and effectively removes the immunity from prosecution which has been enjoyed until now.

Section 2 of the Act provides that for the purpose of health and safety legislation, a health authority shall not be regarded as a servant or agent of the Crown or as enjoying any status, immunity and privilege of the Crown and premises used by a health authority shall not be regarded as property of or property held on behalf of the Crown.

Question 7.1   What statutory controls are in existence in relation to AIDS and HIV infections?

Question 7.2   What justifications can a nurse give for refusing to give care to a patient?
Is Zita's refusal therefore reasonable?
What could be the outcome of Zita's refusal?

Question 7.3   What legal framework should be used to give the nurses support in this situation?
Can you suggest how this could be implemented in practice?

What medical screening for HIV can an employer carry out on prospective or present members of staff?
Is there any legal reason for a nurse with HIV infection to give up her employment?
What precautions should be taken by an Occupational Health Department in relation to maintaining or breaching confidentiality of staff health information?

Question 7.4

Activity 7.1

Find out if your health authority has a control of infection policy. Read the section relevant to AIDS and HIV infection.

Activity 7.2

Does your health authority have a staff policy on health screening for HIV infection?

Once the nurses have been helped to set up the necessary infection control precautions, Lynne, one of the staff nurses, is allocated to care for Alan. She spends some time with him, assessing both his physical and mental condition. His temperature is raised and he has a productive cough. He is very weak and any movement tires him. He also seems very depressed and tells Lynne that he does not think that he has much time left. Lynne leaves him to rest while she completes the admission documentation and collects the equipment he needs in his room.

Two hours later, the doctor arrives to examine Alan and Lynne accompanies him. He diagnoses bronchopneumonia and prescribes antibiotics. Once the doctor has gone Alan tells Lynne that he does not want to prolong his life. As he is going to die anyway, what is the point of taking the antibiotics? Lynne tries to persuade him that it is worth taking the drugs as they will ease his breathing. However not only is Alan adamant that he does not want the drugs but in addition he says to Lynne that if she really wants to help him she could get him some tablets that would 'put him to sleep for ever'. Although Lynne feels very helpless, she quietly explains that she cannot do what he suggests but she will do everything she can to ensure he remains as comfortable as possible. As she leaves the room, Ray arrives. Lynne explains what has just transpired and Ray goes quickly to give what comfort he can to his friend.

Read the material below before answering questions 7.5–7.7. You may also find of use the following answers:

Chapter 1 Nos. 5 and 12
Chapter 4 No. 13
Chapter 5 No. 5
Chapter 6 Nos. 3, 7 and 17

(H) R. *v.* BLAUE 1975

Blaue, the assailant, attacked a woman who was a Jehovah's Witness. She refused consent to the blood transfusion that was necessary to save her life. There was no suggestion that the doctor would have been justified in overriding her refusal of consent.

Blaue was convicted of manslaughter, but acquitted of murder by reason of his diminished responsibility.

Skegg (1984)

(I) SUICIDE ACT 1961

Section 1. The rule of law whereby it is a crime for a person to commit suicide is hereby abrogated.

Section 2(1). A person who aids, abets, counsels or procures the suicide of another or an attempt by another to commit suicide, shall be liable on conviction on indictment to imprisonment.

(J) R. *v.* ADAMS 1957

Dr Adams was charged with the murder of an 81-year-old patient who had suffered a stroke. It was alleged that he had prescribed and administered such large quantities of drugs, especially heroin and morphine, that he must have known the drugs would kill her.

Legal implications of the administration of painkilling drugs which may hasten death was stated by the judge, Devlin J, as follows: 'No people of common sense would say, 'Oh, the doctor caused her death' of an example of a doctor who did or omitted to do something because of which death occurred at 11 o'clock instead of 12 o'clock, or Monday instead of Tuesday. They would say the cause of death was the illness or the injury or whatever it was, which brought her into hospital and the proper medical treatment that is administered and that has an incidental effect of determining the exact moment of death, or may have, is not the cause of death in any sensible use of the term.

If the first purpose of medicine, the restoration of health can no longer be achieved there is still much for a doctor to do, and he is entitled to do all that is proper and necessary to relieve pain and suffering even if the measures he takes may incidentally shorten life'.

Dr Adams was acquitted.

Skegg (1984)

What legal predicaments do the doctor and nurse face when a patient refuses consent to treatment?   *Question 7.5*

Question 7.6   In what circumstances might it be legally acceptable for the doctor or nurse to hasten a patient's death?

Question 7.7   Can the nurse legally take on the role of gaining consent or giving information related to a patient's treatment?

> *Activity 7.3*
> Read the UKCC leaflet on *Exercising Accountability*.

As a result of Alan's wishes not to accept further treatment, the medical staff decide not to take active steps to prolong Alan's life. During the evening his condition deteriorates and he lapses into unconsciousness. The nurses amend his care plan to ensure his safety as well as his comfort. They eventually persuade Ray to go home to get some rest with the promise to call him if there is any change.

At 21.00 hours, the day staff hand over to the night staff, an agency staff nurse, an enrolled nurse and a student. The agency nurse Beryl takes on herself the responsibility of caring for Alan. At 23.30 hours while she is turning him, he arrests. Beryl immediately tells the enrolled nurse to call the arrest team while she initiates resuscitation. The arrest team arrives a few minutes later. They decide not to continue attempts to resuscitate and certify Alan dead. While Beryl accepts the sense of this, she feels a bit put out as there was no record on the nursing notes that the patient was not for resuscitation. She telephones the nursing officer who takes the responsibility for contacting Alan's partner. The nursing officer also advises the staff on laying out Alan's body and what to do about his property. She says that Alan's death may have to be reported to the coroner but reassures Beryl that she has acted quite properly.

Read the material below before answering questions 7.8–7.12. You may also find of use the following answers:

Chapter 1 No. 6
Chapter 5 No. 13
Chapter 6 No. 16

(K) LIVING WILLS: WORKING PARTY REPORT

The Centre for Medical Law and Ethics at King's College London and Age Concern produced a report on living wills in 1988. The following is a summary of the report by Dr David Greaves, a member of the working party which produced it.

There are increasing numbers of incurably ill and incapacitated people, many of whom are elderly, who can be kept alive for prolonged periods by medical treatment and care, but who are incompetent to consent to or refuse such management. In these circumstances the unquestioned application of all possible life-sustaining procedures may not be desired by a majority of the public and is morally debatable. The report covers the medical, ethical and legal issues involved in considering those patients to which this might apply. They are people who have become permanently incompetent in making their wishes known, as a result of terminal illness, serious and permanent illness, disability, or severe dementia.

The term living will refers to a document in which a person, while still competent, requests and directs that certain measures, which may be variously specified, should be adopted if and when he becomes incapable of taking responsibility for his own health care, i.e. by consenting to or refusing treatment. The measures usually relate to the refusal of certain forms of treatment aimed at the preservation of the person's life. A durable (or enduring) power of attorney in the context of health care allows a person, whilst competent, to appoint an agent to act on his behalf, in specified matters of health care, if and when he becomes incompetent.

Journal of Medical Ethics (1988) **14**, 105

(L) LIM *v.* CAMDEN AND ISLINGTON AREA HEALTH AUTHORITY 1979

The patient (herself a doctor) suffered a cardiac arrest after a minor gynaecological operation. Although her breathing and heart beat were eventually restored, her brain had by then suffered severe and irreversible damage. At times she had some memory of the past, could understand a little, read a little and speak a little. At other times she would lapse into a depressed, withdrawn, non-responsive, non-communicative and even non-cooperative behaviour not unlike a child of a few years old. The Health Authority accepted liability for negligence, and the only issue before the courts was the quantum of damages. However in the course of his judgement Lord Denning implied that a doctor was not always obliged to persist in efforts to resuscitate a patient following a cardiac arrest. In this case twenty five minutes had elapsed before the patient's breathing was restored to normal and she was brought back to what Lord Denning described as 'a life which is not worth living'. He said that after an accident such as occurred in this case, those concerned are faced with an agonising decision: is she to be kept alive? Or is she to be allowed to die? Is the thread of life to be maintained to the utmost reach of science? Or should it be let fall and nature take its inevitable course? In such circumstances, those about her should say – 'for mercy's sake, let the end come now.'

Skegg (1984)

(M) CORONERS ACT 1988

The Coroners Act 1988 covers the appointment of coroners, the holding of inquests, and post mortem examination.

Deaths have to be reported to the coroner when:

1. there is reasonable cause to suspect a person has died a violent or unnatural death;
2. there is reasonable cause to suspect a person has died a sudden death of which the cause is unknown;
3. the person has died in prison or in such place or under such circumstances as to require an inquest.

Those causes of death which should be reported to the coroner include: abortions, accidents and injuries, alcoholism, anaesthetics and operations, crime or suspected crime, drugs, ill treatment, industrial diseases, infant deaths if in any way obscure, pensioners where death might be connected with a pensionable disability, persons in legal custody, poisoning, septicaemias if originating from an injury, and stillbirths where there may have been a possibility or suspicion that the child may have been born alive.

Can the patient ensure his wishes are followed regarding acceptance or refusal of medical intervention once he loses consciousness?

Question 7.8

Question 7.9   In what circumstances can the nurse decide not to initiate resuscitation when cardiac arrest occurs?

Question 7.10   What is a legal definition of death?

Question 7.11   What care must be taken of a patient's property at death?

In what circumstances must a death be reported to the coroner? What role may a nurse have to play if this is done?

Activity 7.4

See if there is an opportunity for you to visit a coroner's court.

ANSWERS

Question 7.1

AIDS Control Act 1987
Public Health Act (Infectious Disease) Regulations 1985
National Health Service (Veneral Disease) Regulations 1974 (amended 1982)

Question 7.2

There are very few reasons that a nurse can give for justifying a refusal to care for a patient.

She has a legal right under the Abortion Act 1967 'not to participate in any treatment authorised by this Act to which she has a conscientious objection'. However even this right is limited if treatment is needed 'to save the life or to prevent grave permanent injury to the physical or mental health of a pregnant woman'. It is also quite difficult to differentiate between participation in abortion and the giving of other supportive care when the abortion is taking place on a ward over a number of hours.

The nurse should also refuse to participate if she fears that this would involve her in some criminal activity. For example, if there is an intention to cause the death of a patient by giving certain treatment (see question 7.6), this could be murder or manslaughter.

If she suspects that harm could result to a patient due to some act or omission, this might be negligence. Again, the nurse should avoid being involved. Even if the treatment was authorized by a doctor, the nurse could share the negligence if it was some aspect of care about which she should have had knowledge and experience. The nurse should also refuse to give care if it is beyond her competence to do so as this could also lead to harm to the patient. If the task is appropriate for the nurse to undertake, further training and supervision must then be offered.

Finally if the nurse is asked to participate in care that puts her in danger, she is only justified in refusing until management has responded by providing either facilities to improve her safety or extra training in safety measures. It is this last reason that Zita might argue in refusing to care for Alan but only so long as management failed to act reasonably in the specific circumstances. The provision of a control of infection nursing officer to assist and advise would be considered quite reasonable and Zita would therefore not have sufficient grounds for continuing in her refusal.

An outcome of Zita's continuing refusal would be discipline of some kind. It could be considered that she was in breach of her contract in being selective as to the patients she agreed to nurse and dismissal could therefore follow. She would also have a case to answer to the UKCC professional conduct committee under the Code of Professional Conduct.

Question 7.3

The Health and Safety at Work (etc.) Act 1974 is the main legal framework of use in this circumstance. The employer has a responsibility to give training in the care of patients with AIDS, along with ongoing supervision. This would include information on the mode of transmission of the HIV infection, precautions to take when disposing of body fluids or blood spillages, the exclusion of 'at risk' staff (for example those with cuts or abrasions on the hands) from direct contact with AIDS patients and the prevention of needlestick accidents. The employer also has a responsibility to provide a safe working environment so that provision of protective gloves and aprons, appropriate disinfectants and adequate handwashing facilities would be appropriate. However, the drawback of this legislation is that the employer responsibilities only need to be implemented 'as far as is reasonably practicable' in order to remain within the law.

The employee has a legal duty to cooperate with the employer. Therefore the nursing staff must follow the instructions given when nursing Alan.

Question 7.4

The prospective employer has the right to demand any medical screening of a future employee that is considered appropriate. However, there are legal constraints on discriminatory practices, for example in relation to the Sex Discrimination Act 1975 and the Race Relations Act 1976. Once employment has commenced, the employer must have reasonable grounds for demanding a blood test for HIV. If the employee refuses and is then dismissed, it may be quite difficult for the employer to prove that he had acted reasonably as it seems likely that the employee would have to have been acting in such a way as to recklessly endanger public health. The result of such a blood test is also not conclusive if negative as this does not rule out recent exposure to the virus and frequent testing would therefore be necessary.

In addition, there have been no known cases of a patient contracting the disease from a nurse, and as long as the proper precautions are followed there should be no danger to either patients or fellow employees. Thus there is no reason on either the employer's or employee's part for terminating employment unless sickness levels rise beyond an acceptable amount.

If an Occupational Health Department is involved in such testing, the usual rules of confidentiality should apply. Pre-employment testing would include the collection of other information and the employer need only be told that the candidate is unsuitable for employment on agreed medical grounds. Results of post employment testing should only be divulged with the employee's permission. However, such constraints have no legal authority, giving an employee little redress in law. The Occupational Health Department could argue that a failure to disclose a positive test to the employer could be potential negligence if the employee then acted recklessly or carelessly towards patients or staff. However, as stated above, any employer action in removing or dismissing the employee has little factual basis and the employee might claim unfair dismissal via an industrial tribunal if he has been in employment for two years or more.

Question 7.5

In order for care or treatment to be given the patient must consent or he can sue for assault and battery.

There are several legal predicaments here. The first concerns the patient's capacity to give a valid consent. The patient must have the necessary understanding. Impaired consciousness would clearly render the patient unable to give consent but at this point Alan is fully conscious. If a patient is mentally confused due to the physical effects of the illness, the doctor and nurse would have to proceed without consent on the basis of urgency and necessity. A patient who is mentally ill may occasionally be considered not to have the necessary capacity but any refusal could only be overruled if he is put under section of the Mental Health Act 1983 and any treatment then given must be for the mental illness only. It seems unlikely that Alan's refusal to take the antibiotics can be overruled on either of these grounds. A seemingly irrational refusal can be a competent one, and the doctor and nurse can feel assured that their acceptance of this is legally correct.

A final predicament is a concern that a failure to treat may be interpreted as negligence. As long as the patient's refusal is documented, this fear should be put aside.

Question 7.6

As is stated clearly in the Suicide Act 1961, it is a crime to assist with another person's attempt to commit suicide.

An act that brings about a patient's death may also be murder. However there is one reason or legal defence to exonerate a nurse or doctor in these circumstances. There must usually be the intention to cause death and it may well be that although the giving of a large dose of narcotics, for example, hastens the death of a terminally ill patient, the reason for the drug dose is the relief of pain. For the nurse to feel satisfied as to the motivation of giving a certain drug dose, she should check that the doses have been gradually increased over a period of time, rather than there having been a sudden and massive increase. Such a prescription should be viewed with suspicion.

The law also accepts that care can be omitted when there is no longer any useful purpose to be achieved in continuing with active treatment. In such circumstances, the law will not consider that such omissions constitute negligence. Thus the omission of antibiotics to treat Alan at this point in his illness would probably be acceptable even if Alan had been willing to take them.

Question 7.7

Where it is a question of gaining consent for treatment, this is legally a medical responsibility. However, the nurse can take on certain responsibilities within this constraint. She can ascertain if the patient has understood what the doctor has explained and, if confident of her own knowledge, she can clarify points on which the patient is still unsure. She can assist the patient in asking further questions of the doctor who then has a legal duty to answer them. She can also assist the doctor in assessing how much information the patient wants or if some information may be detrimental to his health.

In other situations involving the giving of information, the responsibility is still the doctor's as he has legal control of knowledge relating to the patient's condition. As above, the nurse can assist the doctor in this role.

However, in all information giving, the nurse must remember that if she gives false or misleading facts, she could be negligent if harm resulted. In situations where the nurse gives correct information to a patient without the doctor's agreement, she may face discipline but it is unlikely that there would be any other legal outcome.

Question 7.8

Once a patient loses the capacity to give a valid consent, as in the loss of consciousness, he cannot expect any previously expressed wishes to be honoured. In any situation, the doctor or nurse has to work on the basis of whether the care is urgently necessary to save life or prevent grave damage. Even if a relative expresses the opinion that the patient would not want certain treatment on religious or other grounds, the professionals have to work on the basis that if the patient could make a decision, he would choose to live rather than to die. However a written expression of the patient's wishes can influence a medical decision, although not control it. For example, while the use of a living will has no legality in this country, it can help to support a medical view that to continue treatment would serve no useful purpose. Another example would be a Jehovah Witness patient undergoing surgery signing a form refusing consent to blood transfusion during the operation. However, an emergency arising during this time could quite legally lead to this document being overruled.

Question 7.9

Legally this is not a decision that a nurse is entitled to make. Thus Beryl acted properly in initiating resuscitation as no medical direction that the patient was not for resuscitation had been recorded. There may be circumstances where the nurse feels sure that this has been an oversight on the part of the doctors. Even so, it is legally advisable to call the arrest team. Once they arrive, the decision not to attempt resuscitation can be theirs. As the Lim case (1979) shows, this can be an acceptable decision.

Question 7.10

A legal definition of death is not as clear as would be supposed. The stoppage of the circulation of the blood and the cessation of the animal and vital functions of the body, such as respiration and pulse, no longer suffice in all situations. The definition of brain stem death has evolved for those patients on life support machines. While this has not been legally tested, in those court cases where life support systems have been discontinued the judges have not queried the medical acceptance of this definition.

Brain stem death involves strict criteria. A range of tests including blood gases, brain stem reflexes and core body temperature have to be carried out at least twice.

Question 7.11

A deceased person's property should be handed over only to the person's executors. Therefore it is important that no property is given to a next of kin or in Alan's case, to his friend. Emotive situations can very quickly arise in relation to a deceased person's property and the nurse is well advised not to get involved. She should closely follow hospital policy, making a list of property and a note of any rings left on the body.

Question 7.12

A death must be reported where there are grounds for suspicion that the death is unnatural or the cause is unknown. In addition there are often specific causes of death that must be reported. The one met most often by the nurse is the patient who dies while under anaesthetic or as a result of an operation. Reporting a death shortly after admission to hospital is not unusual as there may have been insufficient time to confirm a diagnosis.

If a death is reported, the nurse may be required to make a statement of her involvement with the patient. Sometimes, an inquest has to be held. Its purpose is not to apportion blame or guilt, but to determine how, where and when the deceased came by his death. There is rarely a jury. The nurse may have to attend as a witness. She should speak slowly and clearly so that she can be heard. She should use everyday language as far as possible, or, where medical terms have to be used, she should be prepared to explain these. She should avoid abbreviations or jargon and keep to the facts. If she is asked for an opinion, she should make it clear in what capacity she is giving this. Disclosure of confidential information can be legally required, but the nurse should in such situations aim to give the minimum amount of information for the purpose of the hearing.

RELEVANT STATUTES AND CASES

Abortion Act 1967
AIDS Control Act 1987
Coroners Act 1988
Employment Protection (Consolidation) Act 1978
Health and Safety at Work (etc.) Act 1974
Mental Health Act 1983
National Health Service (Amendment) Act 1986
Nurses, Midwives and Health Visitors Act 1979
Public Health Act 1936, amended 1968
Public Health (Control of Diseases) Act 1984
Race Relations Act 1976
Sex Discrimination Act 1975
Suicide Act 1961
Lim *v.* Camden and Islington AHA 1979
R. *v.* Adams 1957
R. *v.* Blaue 1975

REFERENCES

Dimond, B. (1990) *Legal Aspects of Nursing*. Prentice Hall, London.
Greaves, D. (1988) Living Wills: Working Party Report. *Journal of Medical Ethics*, **14**, 105.

Skegg, P.D.G. (1984) *Law, Ethics and Medicine*. Oxford University Press, Oxford.

United Kingdom Central Council (1984) *Code of Professional Conduct*, 2nd edn. UKCC, London.

United Kingdom Central Council (1988) AIDS: testing, treatment and care. *Register*, Jan. 1988. UKCC, London.

United Kingdom Central Council (1988) *AIDS and HIV infection. A UKCC statement*. PC/88/03, March 1988, UKCC, London.

Vousden, M. (1984) Sacked ECT nurse loses appeal. *Nursing Mirror*, **159**, No. 18.

8 Mental health nursing

Bernice lives with her husband and mother-in-law in a first floor flat. She is 28 years old and has been married 5 years. She is a slim woman with long dark hair which she normally wears in a pony tail. Although she has no children, she has not worked since she got married. She is shy and does not mix readily with people, preferring to spend her time at home cooking and cleaning for her husband and mother-in-law.

She has had periods of mental illness in the past, probably from her teens, although her parents have been very protective of her and only occasionally sought medical treatment. Since her marriage she has had little contact with her parents as her husband has had a number of rows with them and will not allow them to visit Bernice at the flat. She has attempted suicide at least twice during this time, once by cutting her wrists and once by trying to climb out of a window. Since this last attempt 3 months ago she has been visited regularly by a community psychiatric nurse (CPN) but this nurse's work with Bernice has been impeded by the mother-in-law whose presence during any interview seems to have driven Bernice totally into her shell. However, the nurse, Sue, is determined to persevere and is eventually rewarded by the mother-in-law displaying enough trust to leave them alone for a short period. She then finds that Bernice seems far from well. She tells Sue that her husband hates her and abuses her, while her mother-in-law is trying to poison her. She goes into some detail of what they are doing to her and Sue suspects that Bernice is experiencing delusions. As Sue is leaving the flat, the mother-in-law follows her and expresses her concern about Bernice who has become increasingly withdrawn over the last two weeks, refuses to talk to her or her son and will not eat with them. She also tells Sue that Bernice is no longer taking her prescribed medication in spite of her pleading with her daughter-in-law to do so. Sue feels so concerned that she contacts the approved social worker and Bernice's GP for further advice. The outcome is the arrangement of Bernice's formal admission to hospital under Section 2 of the Mental Health Act 1983.

Case Studies in Law in Nursing,
Ann P. Young.
Published in 1992 by
Chapman & Hall, London
ISBN 0 412 44130 6.

Read the material below before answering questions 8.1–8.3. You may also find of use the following answers:

Chapter 1 Nos. 4 and 8
Chapter 3 Nos. 5, 7 and 13

(A) MENTAL HEALTH ACT 1983

Part II compulsory admission to hospital and guardianship

Admission for assessment

2.-(1) A patient may be admitted to a hospital and detained for the period allowed by subsection (4) below in pursuance of an application (in this Act referred to as 'an application for admission for assessment') made in accordance with subsections (2) and (3) below.

(2) An application for admission for assessment may be made in respect of a patient on the grounds that –

(a) he is suffering from mental disorder of a nature or degree which warrants the detention of the patient in a hospital for assessment (or for assessment followed by medical treatment) for at least a limited period; and

(b) he ought to be so detained in the interests of his own health or safety or with a view to the protection of other persons.

(3) An application for admission for assessment shall be founded on the written recommendations in the prescribed form of two registered medical practitioners, including in each case a statement that in the opinion of the practitioner the conditions set out in subsection (2) above are complied with.

(4) Subject to the provisions of Section 29(4) below, a patient admitted to hospital in pursuance of an application for admission for assessment may be detained for a period not exceeding 28 days beginning with the day on which he is admitted, but shall not be detained after the expiration of that period unless before it has expired he has become liable to be detained by virtue of a subsequent application, order or direction under the following provisions of this Act.

General provision as to applications

11.-(1) Subject to the provisions of this section, an application for admission for assessment, an application for admission for treatment and a guardianship application may be made either by the nearest relative of the patient or by an approved social worker, and every such application shall specify the qualification of the applicant to make the application.

(2) Every application for admission shall be addressed to the managers of the hospital to which admission is sought and every guardianship application shall be forwarded to the local social services authority named in the application as guardian or, as the case may be, to the local social services authority for the area in which the person so named resides.

(3) Before or within a reasonable time after an application for the admission of a patient for assessment is made by an approved social worker, that social worker shall take such steps as are practicable to

inform the person (if any) appearing to be the nearest relative of the patient that the application is to be or has been made and of the power of the nearest relative under Section 23(2)(a) below.

(4) Neither an application for admission for treatment nor guardianship application shall be made by an approved social worker if the nearest relative of the patient has notified that social worker, or the local social services authority by whom that social worker is appointed, that he objects to the application being made and, without prejudice to the foregoing provision, no such provision shall be made by such a social worker except after consultation with the person (if any) appearing to be the nearest relative of the patient unless it appears to that social worker that in the circumstances such consultation is not reasonably practicable or would involve unreasonable delay.

(5) None of the applications mentioned in subsection (1) above shall be made by any person in respect of a patient unless that person has personally seen the patient within the period of 14 days ending with the date of the application.

General provision as to medical recommendations

12.-(1) The recommendations required for the purposes of an application for the admission of a patient under this Part of this Act (in this Act referred to as 'medical recommendations') shall be signed on or before the date of the application, and shall be given by practitioners who have personally examined the patient either together or separately, but where they have examined the patient separately not more than five days must have elapsed between the days on which the separate examinations took place.

(2) Of the medical recommendations given for the purpose of any such application, one shall be given by a practitioner approved for the purpose of this section by the Secretary of State as having special experience in the diagnosis or treatment of mental disorder: and unless that practitioner has previous acquaintance with the patient, the other such recommendation shall, if practicable, be given by a registered medical practitioner who has such previous acquaintance.

(3) Subject to subsection (4) below, where the application is for the admission of the patient to a hospital which is not a mental nursing home, one (but not more than one) of the medical recommendations may be given by a practitioner on the staff of that hospital, except where the patient is proposed to be accommodated under section 65 or 66 of the National Health Service Act 1977 (which relate to accommodation for private patients).

(4) Subsection (3) above shall not preclude both the medical recommendations being given by practitioners on the staff of the hospital in question if –

(a) compliance with the subsection would result in delay involving serious risk to the health or safety of the patient; and

(b) one of the practitioners giving the recommendations works at the hospital for less than half of the time which he is bound by contract to devote to work in the health service; and

(c) where one of those practitioners is a consultant, the other does not work (whether at the hospital or elsewhere) in a grade in which he is under the consultant's directions.

Duty of approved social workers to make applications for admissions or guardianship

13.-(1) It shall be the duty of an approved social worker to make an application for admission to hospital or a guardianship application in respect of a patient within the area of the local social services authority by which that officer is appointed in any case where he is satisfied that such an application ought to be made and is of the opinion, having regard to any wishes expressed by relatives of the patient or any other relevant circumstances, that it is necessary or proper for the application to be made by him.

(2) Before making an application for the admission of a patient to hospital an approved social worker shall interview the patient in a suitable manner and satisfy himself that detention in a hospital is in all the circumstances of the case the most appropriate way of providing the care and medical treatment of which the patient stands in need.

(3) An application under this section by an approved social worker may be made outside the area of the local social services authority by which he is appointed.

(4) It shall be the duty of a local social services authority, if so required by the nearest relative of a patient residing in their area, to direct an approved social worker as soon as practicable to take the patient's case into consideration under subsection (1) above with a view to making an application for his admission to hospital; and if in any such case that approved social worker decides not to make an application he shall inform the nearest relative of his reasons in writing.

(5) Nothing in this section shall be construed as authorizing or requiring an application to be made by an approved social worker in contravention of the provisions of section 11(4) above, or as restricting the power of an approved social worker to make any application under this Act.

Appointment of approved social workers

114.-(1) A local social services authority shall appoint a sufficient number of approved social workers for the purpose of discharging the functions conferred on them by this Act.

(2) No person shall be appointed by a local social services authority as an approved social worker unless he is approved by the authority as having appropriate competence in dealing with persons who are suffering from mental disorder.

(3) In approving a person for appointment as an approved social worker a local social services authority shall have regard to such matters as the Secretary of State may direct.

Question 8.1   Under what legislation may a patient be legally detained in hospital?

Question 8.2   What specific roles must be played by the approved social worker and the two doctors involved in a Section 2 Order?

Question 8.3   What legal rights must be honoured for the patient being admitted to hospital under Section?
How should the patient be told of her rights?
Can you see any potential difficulties in safeguarding her rights at this time?

Activity 8.1

During your training you will meet community psychiatric nurses (CPNs): Take the opportunity to discuss their roles with them.

Activity 8.2

Look at Forms 2 and 3 of the Mental Health Act 1983 for admission for assessment.

Two critical aspects of Bernice's immediate care are to ensure her safety in view of previous suicide attempts and to give her the prescribed medication. She seems confused and unhappy on admission and expresses the opinion that as her husband no longer wants her, she would be better off dead. For the first two weeks the nurses maintain a fairly close level of supervision, ensuring that she is accompanied to the toilet and the bathroom and does not leave the ward. At the end of this period, Bernice's condition is reviewed. It is felt that she is beginning to respond to treatment, she is more outgoing and she is experiencing fewer paranoid delusions. The level of supervision is therefore decreased, the only proviso being that Bernice must inform the nurses when she is going to have a bath and not leave the ward unaccompanied.

Read the material below before answering questions 8.4–8.6. You may also find of use the following answers:

Chapter 1 No. 8
Chapter 2 Nos. 4, 13 and 15
Chapter 3 Nos. 7 and 12
Chapter 5 No. 5

(B) BOLTON v. STONE 1951

The defendant cricket club was exonerated from liability when a cricket ball was hit out of the cricket ground onto the highway, striking and injuring the plaintiff. The possibility of such an event occurring was clearly foreseeable as balls had been hit from the ground before. But the fact that this had happened only on very rare occasions (six times in 30 years) meant that the risk in the circumstances was one which a reasonable man could appropriately choose not to guard against. Lord Oaksey in Bolton v. Stone opined: 'The standard of care in the law of negligence is the standard of an ordinarily careful man, but in my opinion, an ordinarily careful man does not take precautions against every foreseeable risk. He can, of course, foresee the possibility of many risks, but life would be almost impossible if he were to attempt to take precautions against every risk which he can foresee. He takes precautions against risks which are reasonably likely to happen. Many foreseeable risks are extremely unlikely to happen and cannot be guarded against except by almost complete isolation'.

Tyas (1989)

(C) HEALTH SERVICE COMMISSIONER – SECOND REPORT TO PARLIAMENT FOR SESSION 1988–89 EPITOMES OF SELECTED CASES NOV. 1988–MARCH 1989

Admission, supervision and death of a psychiatric patient

Matters considered

Delay in admitting patient – failure in communication between medical and nursing staff – inadequacy of nursing supervision – return of patient's effects – failure to respond adequately to complaints.

Summary of case

The complainant's brother, who had a history of schizophrenic illness, became agitated and disturbed and the complainant sought to have him admitted direct to the ward on which he had previously been a patient, believing that this had been agreed with the hospital on an earlier occasion. Although he was first directed to the hospital's admissions department the man was subsequently admitted to the ward. The complainant telephoned the hospital later that morning and was told his brother was agitated but that everything was under control. However the man jumped from a window on the ward that afternoon and died as a result of the injuries sustained. The complainant complained that the delay in admitting his brother to the ward caused him to become upset and more agitated. He believed that nursing staff had not been fully informed of the degree of supervision his brother had required and he considered that a patient with a history of jumping from windows should not have been left alone in a room after a window frame had fallen out. He complained that the manner in which his brother's effects were returned to him had caused him great distress and further complained that the meeting he had requested so that his complaints might be more fully discussed was not arranged.

Findings

I was persuaded that the nursing staff were not unduly concerned about the man's condition when he first arrived on the ward and I was also persuaded, given the obvious practical difficulties involved, that it was unlikely that the hospital had entered into any formal agreement with the complainant and/or his family to admit the man direct to the ward. Moreover I did not regard the time taken to admit the man to the ward as unreasonable. I found that considerable time had been spent considering how best to care for the man and I did not accept that there was faulty communication between medical and nursing staff or that the nursing staff were unaware of the problems associated with the man's care. I accepted that they had supervised him correctly during the morning but I learned that he had damaged a window frame in his room during the early part of the afternoon and that the entire frame had fallen out of the room leaving a hole in the wall some four feet by two feet. I saw that the nursing staff believed the medication the man had been given would by then have taken effect but I considered that an error of judgement was made in leaving him unsupervised after the window had fallen out, particularly since it was known that he had jumped from windows previously. I found that the hospital acted wholly insensitively in returning the brother's effects to his family in a blood-stained condition. I considered the hospital's decision to postpone a meeting with the complainant and other members of his family until after the coroner's inquest was reasonable and while I saw that they had made several attempts to contact the complainant by telephone and that the letter they eventually wrote offering a meeting was ignored, I criticized them for not writing to the complainant earlier.

Remedy
The health authority offered their unreserved apologies for the short-comings I identified.

(D) BOLAM v. FRIERN H.M.C. 1957

Mr Bolam agreed to electroconvulsive therapy (ECT) to treat his de-pression. He suffered fractures in the course of the treatment. The risk was known to the doctor but he did not tell Mr Bolam.

Mr Bolam alleged negligence on a number of grounds including the failure to warn him of the risk. The judge found that the amount of information accorded with 'accepted medical practice'. There would only have been negligence if Mr Bolam could have proved that further informa-tion would have led him to refuse consent.

The medical standard of care is the standard of a reasonably skilled and experienced doctor. The judge in the Bolam case stated:

'The test is the standard of the ordinary skilled man exercising and professing to have that special skill. A man need not possess the highest expert skill; it is well established law that it is sufficient if he exercises the ordinary skill of an ordinary competent man exercising that particular art'.

He also added that the doctor had acted 'in accordance with a practice accepted as proper by a responsible body of medical men skilled in that particular area'.

Brazier (1987)

Question 8.4   If Bernice had attempted suicide after admission to hospital, why might the nurses be held to be negligent?

What measures should the nurses take to prevent any suicide attempt?

How much information should the nurses give to Bernice about her medication?

In order to protect themselves from charges of negligence when reducing Bernice's level of supervision, what arguments can the nurses put forward?

Activity 8.3

Find out what safety features are incorporated into the psychiatric ward environment.

After three weeks, Bernice's husband telephones the ward to express the view that his wife should no longer be under Section 2 and that he intends to apply to the Mental Health Review Tribunal for her release. His rights are explained to him. It is also pointed out that a Section 2 order runs for only 28 days and if Bernice's progress continues to be good, the psychiatrist may well decide not to continue to detain her formally. This is what transpires at the end of four weeks and Bernice remains on the ward as an informal patient.

Shortly after a visit from her husband, Bernice is found by one of the nurses in tears. She states that she does not want her husband to visit her as she feels frightened of him. However when he arrives the following day, he insists on seeing his wife and she eventually agrees. After his departure she seems confused and distracted. Later that evening she suddenly pulls a knife from her bag and attacks the nurse sitting beside her. The nurse sustains a badly cut hand before two other nurses come to her assistance, remove the knife from Bernice and physically restrain her. As Bernice's doctor is not immediately available, Section 5 of the Mental Health Act 1983 is invoked.

Read the material below before answering questions 8.7–8.10. You may also find of use the following answers:

Chapter 1 Nos. 5 and 9
Chapter 2 Nos. 11 and 14

(E) MENTAL HEALTH ACT 1983

Restriction on discharge by nearest relative

25.-(1) An order for the discharge of a patient who is liable to be detained in a hospital shall not be made by his nearest relative except after giving not less than 72 hours' notice in writing to the managers of the hospital; and if, within 72 hours after such notice has been given, the responsible medical officer furnishes to the managers a report certifying that in the opinion of that officer the patient, if discharged, would be likely to act in a manner dangerous to other persons or to himself –

(a) any order for the discharge of the patient made by that relative in pursuance of the notice shall be of no effect; and

(b) no further order for the discharge of the patient shall be made by that relative during the period of six months beginning with the date of the report.

(2) In any case where a report under subsection (1) above is furnished in respect of a patient who is liable to be detained in pursuance of an application for admission for treatment the managers shall cause the nearest relative of the patient to be informed.

Definition of 'relative' and 'nearest relative'

26.-(1) In this Part of this Act 'relative' means any of the following persons:

(a) husband or wife;

(b) son or daughter;

(c) father or mother;

(d) brother or sister;

(e) grandparent;

(f) grandchild;

(g) uncle or aunt;

(h) nephew or niece.

(2) In deducing relationships for the purpose of this section, any relationship of the half-blood shall be treated as a relationship of the whole blood, and an illegitimate person shall be treated as the legitimate child of his mother.

(3) In this Part of this Act, subject to the provision of this section and to the following provisions of this Part of this Act, the 'nearest relative' means the person first described in subsection (1) above who is for the time being surviving, relatives of the whole blood being preferred to relatives of the same description of the half-blood and the elder or eldest of two or more relatives described in any paragraph of that subsection being preferred to the other or others of those relatives, regardless of sex.

(F) MENTAL HEALTH ACT 1983

Application in respect of patient already in hospital

5.-(1) An application for the admission of a patient to a hospital may be made under this Part of this Act notwithstanding that the patient is already an in-patient in that hospital or, in the case of an application for admission for treatment that the patient is for the time being liable to be detained in the hospital in pursuance of an application for admission for assessment; and where an application is so made the patient shall be treated for the purposes of this Part of this Act as if he had been admitted to the hospital at the time when that application was received by the managers.

(2) If, in the case of a patient who is an in-patient in a hospital, it appears to the registered medical practitioner in charge of the treatment of the patient that an application ought to be made under this Part of this Act for the admission of the patient to hospital, he may furnish to the managers a report in writing to that effect; and in any such case the patient may be detained in the hospital for a period of 72 hours from the time when the report is furnished.

(3) The registered medical practitioner in charge of the treatment of a patient in a hospital may nominate one (but not more than one) other registered medical practitioner on the staff of that hospital to act for him under subsection (2) above in his absence.

(4) If, in the case of a patient who is receiving treatment for mental disorder as an in-patient in a hospital, it appears to a nurse of the prescribed class –

   (a) that the patient is suffering from mental disorder to such a degree that it is necessary for his health or the protection of others for him to be immediately restrained from leaving the hospital; and

   (b) that it is not practicable to secure the immediate attendance of a practitioner for the purpose of furnishing a report under sub-section (2) above,

the nurse may record that fact in writing; and in that event the patient may be detained in the hospital for a period of six hours from the time when that fact is so recorded or until the earlier arrival at the place where the patient is detained of a practitioner having power to furnish a report under that subsection.

(5) A record made under subsection (4) above shall be delivered by the nurse (or by a person authorized by the nurse on that behalf) to the managers of the hospital as soon as possible after it is made; and where a record is made under that subsection the period mentioned in sub-section (2) above shall begin at the time when it is made.

(G) SOME DEFINITIONS OF CERTAIN CRIMES

Assault (common law offence)

actus reus: an act which causes the victim to fear the immediate application of force against him;

mens rea: an intention to cause the victim to apprehend the immediate application of force or recklessness as to whether the victim might apprehend immediate force.

Battery (common law offence)

actus reus: an act which results in the application of force to the person of another;

mens rea: an intention to apply force or recklessness as to whether force might be applied.

Wounding or causing grievous bodily harm. Section 18 Offences against the Person Act 1861

actus reus: wound or cause any grievous bodily harm to any person;

mens rea: maliciously and unlawfully with intent to do grievous bodily harm or an intent to resist or prevent lawful apprehension or detaining of any person.

Wounding or inflicting grievous bodily harm. Section 20 Offences against the Person Act 1861

actus reus: to wound or inflict any grievous bodily harm upon any other person, either with or without any weapon or instrument;

mens rea: unlawfully and maliciously (intentional or recklessly and without lawful justification).

Dimond (1990)

(H) THE McNAGHTEN RULES

The definition of insanity as a defence is based on the McNaghten Rules, which were laid down in 1843. The basic propositions are:

> every man is presumed to be sane and to possess a sufficient degree of reason to be responsible for his crimes, until the contrary be proved:

> and that to establish a defence on ground of insanity, it must be clearly proved that at the time of the committing of the act, the party accused was labouring under such a defect of reason, from disease of mind, as not to know the nature and quality of the act he was doing, or if he did know it, that he did not know he was doing what was wrong.

Dimond (1990)

(I) CRIMINAL JUSTICE ACT 1988

Compensation from the criminal injuries board

Compensation for personal injury (which includes any disease, any harm to a person's physical or mental condition and pregnancy) is payable if it is a criminal injury, i.e. caused by a specified offence of violence (including arson and trespass on a railway) or caused by the apprehension of an offender or suspected offender, the prevention of the commission of an offence or assisting a constable in such activities.

Compensation can be made for the injury, any loss or damage of property, for funeral expenses, to dependents following a death, for rape and for the birth of a child conceived as a result of rape.

The claimant must satisfy the Board that he took all reasonable steps within a reasonable time to inform the police or other appropriate authority and has given appropriate assistance, and that there is no possibility that the person responsible for causing the injury will benefit from an award.

Question 8.7 What rights do relatives have in appealing against the formal detention of their next of kin?

Question 8.8 What role does the nurse play when a patient refuses to see a visitor?

Section 5 of the Mental Health Act 1983 gives the nurse a legal hold-ing power of the informal patient when a doctor is not immediately available. How must this be carried out?

Question 8.9

_____
Question 8.10   What legal redress might the injured nurse be able to get? Why might
_____   she feel constrained in taking legal action?

Activity 8.4
Study the relevant MHA forms.

Three months later, Bernice is not experiencing any delusions and is
functioning independently. She is considered fit to go home as long as
she continues to take her medications and attends the outpatient
department on a regular basis.

Read the material below before answering question 8.11.

(J) MENTAL HEALTH ACT 1983

Effect of guardianship application, etc.

8.-(1) Where a guardianship application, duly made under the provisions of this Part of this Act and fowarded to the local social services authority within the period allowed by subsection (2) below is accepted by that authority, the application shall, subject to regulations made by the Secretary of State, confer on the authority or person named in the application as guardian, to the exclusion of any other person –

(a) the power to require the patient to reside at a place specified by the authority or person named as guardian;

(b) the power to require the patient to attend at places and times so specified for the purpose of medical treatment, occupation, education or training;

(c) the power to require access to the patient to be given, at any place where the patient is residing, to any registered medical practitioner, approved social worker or other person so specified.

Leave of absence from hospital

17.-(1) The responsible medical officer may grant to any patient who is for the time being liable to be detained in a hospital under this Part of this Act leave to be absent from the hospital subject to such conditions (if any) as that officer considers necessary in the interests of the patient or for the protection of other persons.

(2) Leave of absence may be granted to a patient under this section either indefinitely or on specified occasions or for any specified period; and where leave is so granted for a specified period, that period may be extended by further leave granted in the absence of the patient.

(3) Where it appears to the responsible medical officer that it is necessary so to do in the interests of the patient or for the protection of other persons, he may, upon granting leave of absence under this section, direct that the patient remain in custody during his absence; and where leave of absence is so granted the patient may be kept in the custody of any officer on the staff of the hospital, or of any other person authorized in writing by the managers of the hospital or, if the patient is required in accordance with conditions imposed on the grant of leave of absence to reside in another hospital, of any officer on the staff of that other hospital.

(4) In any case where a patient is absent from a hospital in pursuance of leave of absence granted under this section, and it appears to the responsible medical officer that it is necessary so to do in the interests of the patient's health or safety or for the protection of other persons, that officer may, subject to subsection (5) below, by notice in writing given to the patient or to the person for the time being in charge of

the patient, revoke the leave of absence and recall the patient to the hospital.

(5) A patient to whom leave of absence is granted under this section shall not be recalled under subsection (4) above after he has ceased to be detained under this Part of the Act; and without prejudice to any other provision of this Part of the Act any such patient shall cease to be so liable at the expiration of the period of six months beginning with the first day of his absence on leave unless either –

(a) he has returned to the hospital, or has been transferred to another hospital under the following provision of this Act, before the expiration of that period; or

(b) he is absent without leave at the expiration of that period.

Question 8.11   What measures can be taken to ensure Bernice's compliance to the discharge requirements?

ANSWERS

Question 8.1

1. Under the appropriate section of the Mental Health Act 1983.
2. By means of a magistrate's order under the Public Health Act 1936 or the National Assistance Act 1948.

Question 8.2

The local authority employs a number of approved social workers to implement the relevant parts of the Mental Health Act 1983. The approved social worker has to undergo specific training that is recognized and assessed or he must have appropriate experience in dealing with mentally disordered people before the local authority will proceed with the appointment.

The approved social worker has to follow certain steps in making an application for admission of a patient to hospital under Section. If the approach to the social services department has been made by a relative the social worker has a duty to follow this up as soon as is practicable. He must interview the patient and satisfy himself that detention in hospital is the most appropriate way of providing care. There is an additional duty for the approved social worker to inform the nearest relative of the application.

The other requirement for admission of the patient under Section is the completion of medical recommendations. These must be completed and signed on or before the date of the application. One of the two registered medical practitioners required under Section 2 must have special experience in the diagnosis and treatment of mental disorder. If practicable, one of the doctors should have had previous acquaintance with the patient. The patient must have been examined within the period of 14 days prior to admission.

Question 8.3

The patient has the following rights:

1. to be told the conditions of the detention in hospital regarding period of time and reasons;
2. to be told what the patient can do if she wishes to leave hospital during the period of the detention by applying to the hospital managers or the Mental Health Review Tribunal;
3. to know what conditions have to be met when the doctor orders treatment for the patient's disorder, including the special conditions applying to certain rare treatments and electroconvulsive therapy;
4. to complain to or ask for help from the Mental Health Act Commission;
5. to receive and send letters unless a person has specifically stated that he does not want to receive letters from the patient;
6. to understand the potential involvement of the patient's nearest relative and the right not to have the nearest relative informed.

The patient should be informed both orally and in writing. Special leaflets informing patients of their rights under each Section are printed by HMSO.

There may be some difficulties in ensuring a patient's rights are safeguarded over the period of compulsory admission. In Bernice's case, she may be so severely affected by her paranoid delusions that she cannot understand the implications of what is being explained. Sometimes mental illness can make a patient very apathetic and therefore lacking the will to take action against the detention or to refuse certain treatments. Although treatment for the mental disorder can be given without Bernice's consent during the 28 days of the detention, there is the temptation that if treatment is needed for some conditions *not* causing the mental disorder, this is still given without consent. Although there is always the right to complain to the Mental Health Act Commission, this may be seen by the patient as part of the establishment and therefore not impartial in safeguarding patient's rights.

Question 8.4

Bernice had attempted suicide before although not during the present episode of her illness and she is also expressing possible suicidal thoughts. The nurses must therefore accept the increased likelihood of her taking this course of action compared to another patient who had no such history. As illustrated in Bolton v. Stone 1951 negligence has to be linked to 'sufficient probability' and a reasonable nurse should anticipate the risk. However, there could be some argument as to how probable was a suicide attempt. The nurses are best advised to err on the safe side by taking a number of precautions. Bernice should be observed at frequent intervals, she should not be allowed alone into areas of potential danger such as the bathroom or kitchen and her property should be checked for items that might be used in a suicide attempt such as tablets, scarf or belt. The security of the environment should also be maintained, for example with locked windows and shatterproof glass.

Question 8.5

In law the only way to quantify the amount of information that a patient should be given about treatment is to measure this against accepted medical practice. Redress for inadequate information could involve suing for negligence if the patient can prove that this failure led him to consent to treatment he would otherwise have refused. Accepted practice here means the amount of information accepted as being sufficient 'by a responsible body of medical men skilled in that particular area' (Bolam v. Friern H.M.C. 1957).

In Bernice's case the legal situation is modified by the fact that the medication can be given without her consent as she is being formally detained and is within the first three months of this detention. The nurses might agree that as her consent is not needed, there is no requirement to give her information about her treatment. However this would scarcely be good care on other grounds, although the nurses will have to judge the right amount of information to give in order to promote cooperation without causing the patient distress.

Question 8.6

The nurses need to use a risk assessment strategy, weighing up the likelihood of good or harm resulting from increasing Bernice's independence compared to the possible good or harm if close supervision is continued. As Bernice's mental state improves, the possibility of her harming herself becomes less although does not disappear altogether. Increasing independence therefore becomes less risky although Bernice may initially find it difficult to take on responsibility for her actions. The good of Bernice learning to function effectively can also be weighed against the value of maintaining safety in a very protected environment.

The decision to reduce supervision and encourage independence must be shown to be a reasonable one.

Question 8.7

Under the Mental Health Act 1983, the term 'nearest relative' has special significance as this person has certain rights and responsibilities. He can write to the hospital managers requesting them to let the patient leave. 72 hours notice must be given for them to consider the request on consultation with the doctor. A patient detained under Section 2 can himself apply for discharge within the first 14 days to the Mental Health Review Tribunal but the nearest relative can only do so if the doctor has barred the relative's request to the hospital managers.

Question 8.8

A visitor cannot insist on seeing a patient against his will. Bernice's husband would become a trespasser if he entered the ward after he had been asked to leave by the staff. Thus the nurses have an important role to play in reinforcing the patient's wishes by making the situation clear to the visitor concerned. Of course, the nurses may be of the opinion that Bernice's unwillingness to see her husband has no logical basis and it is part of their role to discuss her feelings with her in the expectation that she might change her mind.

Question 8.9

1. The patient must be suffering from a mental disorder to such a degree that it is necessary for his health and safety or for the protection of others to restrain him from leaving hospital when the doctor responsible is not immediately available.
2. The nurse taking on this power must be registered either as a mental nurse or a mental handicap nurse.
3. She must record when the holding power starts on the prescribed form (No. 13) and this must be delivered to the hospital managers as soon as possible.
4. If the responsible medical officer does not arrive within the 6 hours maximum specified by the Act, the nurse must inform the managers that the holding power has lapsed.

The usual outcome of the nurse undertaking this holding power is for the doctor to formally detain the patient when he arrives using Form 12. The Mental Health Act 1983 gives no further guidance on how the holding power is to be implemented, but most hospitals have their own policies. Under common law the nurses can use reasonable force in self defence or the defence of others.

Question 8.10

The nurse cannot expect the police to prosecute Bernice for wounding or inflicting grievous bodily harm under the Offences Against the Person Act 1861 as the plea of insanity is likely to be accepted. Similarly, a prosecution for assault and battery would also fail as Bernice lacks the necessary intention. However, the nurse should still inform the police of the attack and complete a statement. This could be useful if at a later date she wished to claim compensation from the Criminal Injuries Board.

The employer has a duty to provide a safe system of working but in this instance it would be difficult to ascertain that there was negligence on the part of the employer in enabling Bernice to get hold of a knife. The employer only has to take reasonable precautions. Under the Health and Safety at Work (etc.) Act 1974, the employer has to provide training, for example in the management of violence. A failure to do so would be cause for complaint and possibly negligence, but again quite minimal training may well be considered sufficient.

The nurse can sue the patient herself. Assault and battery are civil wrongs as well as crimes, but in a civil court intention does not have to be proved. Thus Bernice would be liable in spite of her mental state. However, the nurse is deterred from taking this action for two reasons. First, even if she wins the case, she may not benefit financially as the patient may not have the money to pay the compensation awarded. Secondly, many nurses feel unwilling to sue a patient who has been in their care as they feel they have a responsibility towards and a relationship with the patient which they are unwilling to destroy.

Question 8.11

There are two possible ways of attempting to ensure Bernice's compliance to her treatment. The doctor could keep Bernice under Section but grant her leave of absence and this could run for as long as 6 months. A failure by Bernice to take her medication or attend the outpatient department could then lead to a withdrawal of her leave and her return to hospital. However, most professionals would be of the opinion that to try to ensure compliance by means of such a powerful threat is not satisfactory.

Guardianship may be considered. The local social services department usually takes on this role (rarely the nearest relative) and can require attendance at specified places for medical treatment. However the guardian cannot enforce these provisions nor the taking of medication. The guardianship role is therefore very limited in these particular circumstances.

Bernice's compliance to her treatment once she leaves hospital cannot therefore be ensured by law.

RELEVANT STATUTES AND CASES

Criminal Justice Act 1988
Health and Safety at Work (etc.) Act 1974
Hospital Complaints Procedure Act 1985
Mental Health Act 1983
National Assistance Act 1948
National Health Service Act 1977
Offences Against the Person Act 1861
Public Health Act 1936
Bolam *v.* Friern H.M.C. 1957
Bolton *v.* Stone 1951

REFERENCES

Brazier, M. (1987) *Medicine, Patients and the Law*. Penguin, Harmondsworth, Middlesex.

Department of Health (1989) *Report of the Health Service Commissioner, Second Report to Parliament of Session 1988–89, Epitomes of Selected Cases November 1988–March 1989*. Dept. of Health, London.

Department of Health and Welsh Office (1990) *Code of Practice, Mental Health Act 1983*. HMSO, London.

Dimond, B. (1990) *Legal Aspects of Nursing*. Prentice Hall, London.

Jones, R. (1985) *Mental Health Act Manual*. Sweet and Maxwell, London.

Royal College of Nursing (1979) *Seclusion and Restraint in Hospitals and Units for the Mentally Disordered*. R.C.N., London.

Tyas, J.G.M. (1977) *Law of Torts*, 5th edn. M and E Handbooks, McDonald and Evans Ltd., Plymouth.

Whitehead, T. (1983) *Mental Illness and the Law*. Blackwell, Oxford.

9 Mental handicap nursing

Carl is 25 years old. He has severe learning difficulties due to Down's syndrome. Until recently he has been living with his parents, his father being 73 years old and his mother 68 years old. Three months ago his father died after a short illness. Since then his mother has found it increasingly difficult to look after Carl who has responded badly to his father's death with regression to very childish and antisocial behaviour. A place is found for Carl in a small unit for six mentally handicapped adults and two resident members of staff.

Initially Carl is very unsettled. He has frequent temper tantrums and is verbally abusive towards the other members of this small community. His table manners are poor and he refuses to take on tasks around the house. As he is a well built and strong young man, several of the residents are frightened by Carl's behaviour in case it escalates into physical violence. The staff contact Carl's GP who prescribes tranquillizers for a short period. However, Carl refuses to take these. Pat, a registered mental handicap nurse who comes to the house daily, decides instead to draw up a detailed plan of care to help Carl with support, rewards for good behaviour and a full timetable of constructive activities. With Pat's help this is implemented by John an enrolled nurse, and Annabel a care worker, the two resident staff members.

Read the material below before answering questions 9.1–9.3. You may also find of use the following answers:

Chapter 1 No. 12
Chapter 3 No. 14
Chapter 4 No. 3
Chapter 5 Nos. 1 and 2

(A) THE CHRONICALLY SICK AND DISABLED PERSONS ACT 1970

3.-(1) Every local authority for the purposes of Part V of the Housing Act 1957 in discharging their duty under section 91 of that Act to consider housing conditions in their district and the needs of the district with

Case Studies in Law and Nursing,
Ann P. Young.
Published in 1992 by
Chapman & Hall, London
ISBN 0 412 44130 6.

respect to the provision of further housing accommodation shall have regard to the special needs of chronically sick or disabled persons; and any proposals prepared and submitted to the Minister by the authority under that section for the provision of new houses shall distinguish any houses which the authority propose to provide which make special provision for the needs of such persons.

(2) In the application of this section to Scotland for the words 'Part V of the Housing Act 1957', '91' and 'Minister' there shall be substituted respectively by the words 'Part VII of the Housing (Scotland) Act 1966', '137' and 'Secretary of State'.

(B) T *v.* T. 1988

The defendant was a woman aged 19 who was epileptic and severely mentally handicapped. She was totally dependent upon others and was cared for by her mother. She became pregnant and termination of pregnancy was recommended by the medical advisers on the ground that it would be impossible for her to understand the concept of pregnancy or to cope with the difficulties and complications associated with that condition, and that she would be incapable of providing and caring for a child. The doctors also recommended that she should be protected from any further pregnancies by being sterilized. The doctors were, however, unwilling to carry out the abortion or sterilization operation without authorization. The mother thus applied to the court for a declaration that the procedures could be carried out lawfully.

The court held that the situation was not covered by the Mental Health Act 1983 consent to treatment provisions, nor did a guardian under the Act have the power to give consent. They also held that the court no longer had its power to act as *parens patriae* (a kind of wardship jurisdiction) and the court could therefore not give consent itself. (It held that this power had been repealed in 1959 and should be reinstated.) However, the Court was prepared to grant the declaration requested and declared the proposed treatment lawful and therefore a defence to any action for trespass to the person. The doctors would be carrying out the treatment in the interests of the patient as part of their duty of care to the patient.

Dimond (1990)

(C) F. *v.* WEST BERKSHIRE HEALTH AUTHORITY 1989

In this case the court had to decide whether the sterilization of a mentally handicapped woman F aged 35 would be unlawful because of her lack of capacity to give her consent to the operation. Mr Justice Scott Baker in the Family Division granted a declaration that it was in the best interests of F to have the operation. He stated that there was a problem when because of a mental condition a patient was unable to give any meaningful consent to treatment for a physical condition. A doctor if he did nothing could be said to be negligent, if he operated he, *prima facie*, committed the tort of battery. The law's answer to this was that a professional was not liable if he acted in good faith and in the best interests of the patients. The Court of Appeal upheld this decision. The House of Lords (1989 2 All ER 545) confirmed the power at common law for a doctor to act in the best interests of the patient incapable of giving consent. The court also had an inherent jurisdiction to make declarations on the lawfulness of such treatment. Court involvement in cases of sterilization was highly desirable as a matter of good practice.

Dimond (1990)

Question 9.1

What are the responsibilities of the local authority regarding the provision of homes for the mentally handicapped?

What legal issues are raised by Carl's refusal to consent to medication?   *Question 9.2*

Section 18A of the Nurses Rules identifies 13 outcomes that must be achieved for entry to the Register. Which of these are demonstrated by Pat?   *Question 9.3*

John, who has been working in this house for the last 6 months, is asked to take on particular responsibilities for Carl. Over the next few days, Carl continues to be uncooperative and he remains sullen when John suggests various activities. However John notices that Carl has started talking to the resident cat and by the second day when John asks Carl to give the cat its dinner, he is eager to do so. Carl tips the whole contents of a can of catfood onto the dish. When John explains that this is too much for the cat, Carl suddenly turns on him and tells him to _____ off. This is the last straw for John who has found the last 18 hours extremely frustrating. He shouts back at Carl who in response hurls the empty can across the kitchen. John then loses his temper and pushes Carl hard to get him out of the kitchen. Carl is caught off balance and falls awkwardly, banging his head on a cupboard unit. Hearing the raised voices, Annabel rushes into the kitchen as this happens. She checks that Carl is not badly hurt although his forehead is bruised and suggests he sits quietly watching television with one of the other residents. Later that evening, Carl's mother visits her son.

Read the material below before answering questions 9.4 and 9.5. You may also find of use the following answers:

Chapter 3 No. 18
Chapter 5 No. 10
Chapter 6 No. 4

Material in Chapter 8 is also relevant.

(D) UKCC PROFESSIONAL CONDUCT COMMITTEE HEARING

A divisional nursing officer for a large mental handicap division brought to the Council allegations concerning an RNMH aged 31 years.

It was alleged that the woman (who had been in the employment of the particular hospital for 11 years) had hit a child on the head with her shoe, and that she had submitted an accident form which misrepresented the facts as they subsequently emerged.

At the Committee the first witness was a nursing assistant (an intelligent young married woman who had been employed for 9 months). She was in charge of a ward for active mentally handicapped children at night and had been told to keep a special eye on a boy called Tommy. He began to play up and as she was anxious about the situation, and this was the first time she had been on this ward, she went to the adjacent ward to ask the trained nurse there for guidance. The nurse (the subject of the case) went to the nursing assistant's ward half an hour later, and helped her to cope with the situation and put the children to bed. The last was a boy named Philip. Shortly after this Philip got out of bed (which he had wet) and stripped it. The witness alleged that the nurse concerned took hold of Philip, smacked him on the face and body with the palm of her hand about 12 times, and then took her right shoe off. With that shoe she struck Philip a number of blows; one was a hard blow on top of the head. Philip then broke free and ran to hide behind a locker. The witness comforted the child and found that his face was covered with blood. The nurse took Philip to the bathroom, bathed his face, and located the cut. The nurse then said to the witness that she would have to report the matter, but it would be better to say that the child cut his head on the locker. She asked the witness to cover her if she said that. The witness was relatively inexperienced, and at first said that she would.

The doctor came and treated the wound. He signed the accident report on which it was stated that Philip had fallen and hit the corner of the locker. The witness thought the matter over, and when she was next on duty (4 days later) she reported the incident.

The second witness was the doctor (a registrar). He said that at about 10.30 pm he received a call from the ward and went as requested. Philip was brought to him and he found that there was a jagged laceration on the top of his head. This jagged wound was said to be about 4 cm long. He cleaned the wound, sutured it and applied a dressing. He then completed the partly filled accident form. The third witness was the divisional nursing officer. He gave evidence that having received a report from the nursing assistant, he interviewed the nurse in the presence of her union representative. The nurse admitted that she had contacted the patient with her shoe, but insisted that she had not struck the patient. He was told that she took the new shoe off because it was hurting her, and Philip rubbed his head against it. She admitted that she had submitted a false accident form. In consequence, the divisional nursing officer dismissed the nurse concerned, though in this evidence he did confirm that she had been in the employment of his division (as student and trained nurse) for 11 years, and there had been no previous cause for concern.

In her evidence the nurse insisted that she had taken her shoe off because it was hurting her, and that while she had it in her hand Philip ran into her and rubbed his head against the heel. She admitted that the evidence concerning the cover-up was true and that the accident report was false, but she said that she had submitted false particulars as she was 'shocked at what I had accidently caused and I panicked'. She argued that never had she ever either knowingly or accidentally caused harm to a patient.

The Committee were satisfied that the allegations were proved, and that the facts constituted professional misconduct.

The decision was made to remove her name from the Register.

Pyne (1981)

(E) NURSES, MIDWIVES AND HEALTH VISITORS ACT 1979

2.-(1) The principal functions of the Central Council shall be to establish and improve standards of training and professional conduct for nurses, midwives and health visitors.

(2) The Council shall ensure that the standards of training they establish are such as to meet any Community obligation of the United Kingdom.

(3) The Council shall by means of rules determine the conditions of a person's being admitted to training, and the kind and standard of training to be undertaken, with a view to registration.

(4) The rules may also make provision with respect to the kind and standard of further training available to persons who are already registered.

(5) The powers of the Council shall include that of providing, in such manner as it thinks fit, advice for nurses, midwives and health visitors on standards of professional conduct.

(6) In the discharge of its functions the Council shall have proper regard for the interests of all groups within the professions, including those with minority representation.

12.-(1) The Central Council shall by rules determine circumstances in which, and the means by which –

(a) a person may, for misconduct or otherwise, be removed from the register or a part of it, whether or not for a specified period;

(b) a person who has been removed from the register or a part of it may be restored to it; and

(c) an entry in the register may be removed, altered or restored.

(2) Committees of the Council shall be constituted by the rules to hear and determine proceedings for a person's removal from, or restoration to, the register or for the removal, alteration or restoration of any entry.

(3) The committee shall be constituted from members of the Council; and the rules shall so provide that the members of a committee constituted to adjudicate upon the conduct of any person are selected with due regard to the professional field in which that person works.

(4) The rules shall make provision as to the procedure to be followed, and the rules of evidence to be observed, in such proceedings, whether before the Council itself or before any committee so constituted, and for the proceedings to be in public except in such cases (if any) as the rules may specify.

(5) Schedule 3 to this Act has effect with respect to the conduct of proceedings to which this section applies.

13.-(1) A person aggrieved by a decision to remove him from the register, or to remove or alter any entry in respect of him, may, within 3 months after the date on which notice of the decision is given to him by the Council, appeal to the appropriate court; and on the appeal –

(a) the court may give such directions in the matter as it thinks proper, including directions as to the costs of the appeal; and

(b) the order of the court shall be final.

(2) The appropriate court for the purposes of this section is the High Court, the Court of Session or the High Court in Northern Ireland, according as the appellant's ordinary place of residence is in England or Wales, Scotland or Northern Ireland at the time when notice of the decision is given.

(F) EMPLOYMENT PROTECTION (CONSOLIDATION) ACT 1978

Right of employee not to be unfairly dismissed

54.-(1) In every employment to which this section applies every employee shall have the right not to be unfairly dismissed by his employer.

(2) This section applies to every employment except in so far as its application is excluded by or under any provision of this Part or by sections 141 to 149.

Meaning of 'dismissal'

55.-(1) In this Part, except as respects a case to which section 56 applies, 'dismissal' and 'dismiss' shall be construed in accordance with the following provisions of this section.

(2) Subject to subsection (3), an employee shall be treated as dismissed by his employer if, but only if, –

   (a) the contract under which he is employed by the employer is terminated by the employer, whether it is so terminated by notice or without notice, or

   (b) where under that contract he is employed for a fixed term, that term expires without being renewed under the same contract, or

   (c) the employee terminates that contract, with or without notice in circumstances such that he is entitled to terminate it without notice by reason of the employer's conduct.

(3) Where an employer gives notice to an employee to terminate his contract of employment and, at a time within the period of that notice, the employee gives notice to the employer to terminate the contract of employment on a date earlier than the date on which the employer's notice is due to expire, the employee shall for the purpose of this Part be taken to be dismissed by his employer, and the reasons for the dismissal shall be taken to be the reasons for which the employer's notice is given.

General provision relating to fairness of dismissal

57.-(1) In determining for the purpose of this Part whether the dismissal of an employee was fair or unfair, it shall be for the employer to show –

   (a) what was the reason (or, if there was more than one, the principal reason) for the dismissal, and

   (b) that it was a reason falling within subsection (2) or some other substantial reason of a kind such as to justify the dismissal of an employee holding the position which that employee held.

(2) In subsection (1)(b) the reference to a reason falling within this subsection is a reference to a reason which –

   (a) related to the capability or qualifications of the employee for performing work of the kind which he was employed by the employer to do, or

   (b) related to the conduct of the employee, or

   (c) was that the employee was redundant, or

   (d) was that the employee could not continue to work in the position which he held without contravention (either on his part or on that of his employer) of a duty or restriction imposed by or under an enactment.

(3) Where the employer has fulfilled the requirements of subsection (1), then, subject to sections 58 and 62, the determination of the question whether the dismissal was fair or unfair, having regard to the reason shown by the employer, shall depend on whether the employer can satisfy the tribunal that in the circumstances (having regard to equity and the substantial merits of the case) he acted reasonably in treating it as a sufficient reason for dismissing the employee.

(4) In this section, in relation to an employee, –

(a) 'capability' means capability assessed by reference to skill, aptitude, health or any other physical or mental quality;

(b) 'qualifications' means any degree, diploma or other academic, technical or professional qualification relevant to the position which the employee held.

Complaint to industrial tribunal

67.-(1) A complaint may be presented to an industrial tribunal against an employer by any person (in this Part referred to as the complainant) that he was unfairly dismissed by the employer.

(2) Subject to subsection (4), an industrial tribunal shall not consider a complaint under this section unless it is presented to the tribunal before the end of the period of three months beginning with the effective date of termination or within such further period as the tribunal considers reasonable in a case where it is satisfied that it was not reasonably practicable for the complaint to be presented before the end of the period of three months.

Remedies for unfair dismissal

68.-(1) Where on a complaint under section 67 an industrial tribunal finds that the grounds of the complaint are well-founded, it shall explain to the complainant what orders for reinstatement or re-engagement may be made under section 69 and in what circumstances they may be made, and shall ask him whether he wishes the tribunal to make such an order, and if he does express such a wish the tribunal may make an order under section 69.

(2) If on a complaint under section 67 the tribunal finds that the grounds for the complaint are well-founded and no order is made under section 69, the tribunal shall make an award of compensation for unfair dismissal, calculated in accordance with sections 72 to 74, to be paid by the employer to the employee.

Question 9.4   Why does John's action against Carl constitute battery? List the possible outcomes to John of his action.

If dismissal follows, does he have any right of appeal?

If Carl's mother wanted to make a complaint, how would she go about this?   *Question 9.5*

Activity 9.1

Find out the procedures followed by the UKCC when a case of alleged misconduct is reported to it.

Activity 9.2

Ask your tutor if it is possible to arrange a visit to either a UKCC professional conduct committee hearing or an industrial tribunal.

Carl gradually settles down and starts participating in the activities of the home. He makes friends with several of the residents. Lizzie is feeling pleased with herself as she has just got a part-time job in the nearby supermarket. She helps with stacking shelves and enjoys working with and meeting new people. Billy is taking a cookery course at college and hopes that this might lead to a job although for the time being he is experimenting on his 'family' in the house. Damien, who is physically as well as mentally handicapped, also enjoys Carl's company and Carl spends some time choosing what music to play for him from his collection of tapes.

Every month, the residents hold a meeting to discuss issues concerning the running of the house. Several months after Carl's arrival, one of these meetings is scheduled and several issues lead to heated discussion. A complaint is made that some members are failing to do their share of the chores. Lizzie is particularly blamed but claims she is too tired now she is working. As the others refuse to accept this, she says she is going to try to move out into her own place. The issue of money and resources also gets an airing. Carl would like a colourful rug in his room and some of the others agree that they would all like rugs around the house to make it brighter. Pat, who always attends these meetings, says that she will explore the availability of funds for this. A suggestion from Billy that they have a party then effectively terminates discussion of other issues. The party rapidly escalates into a banquet, and the original idea for a small gathering also snowballs into something bigger. Eventually as the arguments seem to be getting out of hand, Annabel brings them back to the practicalities and persuades them to plan a reasonably small and simple event for next week.

Read the material below before answering questions 9.6–9.10. You may also find of use the following answers:

Chapter 2 Nos. 13 and 15
Chapter 3 No. 13

Chapter 4 No. 7
Chapter 5 Nos. 6 and 18

There is also relevant material in Chapter 8.

(G) EDUCATION ACT 1981

(Came into force April 1983)

Main provisions

1. The categories of different types of handicap are abolished and replaced by one of special educational need.
2. LEAs have a duty to provide special educational provision in ordinary schools provided this is compatible with:
   (a) receiving the necessary special provision;
   (b) the efficient education of other children;
   (c) the efficient use of resources.
3. Governors have a duty to ensure that all children in their schools, whether special or ordinary, with special educational needs are having those needs met.
4. LEAs have a duty to identify and assess those children for whom they are responsible who have, or probably have special educational needs. If as a result of the assessment the LEA is of the opinion that special educational provision is necessary, it makes a statement of the child's needs.
5. Parents must be informed of the assessment and can make written representations to it. They can appeal against the statement of needs.
6. If District Health Authorities consider that a child under five has special educational needs they have a duty to inform the parents and the LEA. They must also tell parents of any voluntary organizations that may be able to help them.
7. Children under two with special needs may be assessed with the consent, or at the request, of the parents.

(H) NATIONAL HEALTH SERVICE AND COMMUNITY CARE ACT 1990

Part III – Community Care: England and Wales

Section 42 enables local authorities to provide care for expectant and nursing mothers and to make arrangements for nursing home care in private and voluntary homes; replaces spent provisions enabling local authorities to make arrangements with persons carrying on private and voluntary homes; enables authorities to employ voluntary organizations and private concerns as their agents in the provision of welfare services; and provides an alternative method of payment for use when accommodation is arranged with housing associations.

(I) EMPLOYMENT PROTECTION (CONSOLIDATION) ACT 1978

Changes in terms of employment

4.-(4) Where, after an employer has given to an employee a written statement in accordance with section 1 –

(a) the name of the employer (whether an individual or a body corporate or partnership) is changed, without any change in the identity of the employer, or

(b) the identity of the employer is changed, in such circumstances that, in accordance with section 139 (7) or paragraph 17 or paragraph 18 of Schedule 13, the continuity of the employee's period of employment is not broken,

and (in either case) the change does not involve any change in the terms (other than the names of the parties) included or referred to in the statement, then, the person who, immediately after the change, is the employer shall not be required to give to the employee a statement in accordance with section 1, but, subject to subsection (5), the change shall be treated as a change falling within subsection (1) of this section.

(5) A written statement under this section which informs an employee of such a change in his terms of employment as is referred to in subsection (4)(b) shall specify the date on which the employee's continuous period of employment began.

Renewal of contract or re-engagement

84.-(1) If an employee's contract of employment is renewed, or he is re-engaged under a new contract of employment in pursuance of an offer (whether in writing or not) made by his employer before the ending of his employment under the previous contract, and the renewal or re-engagement takes effect either immediately on the ending of that employment or after an interval of not more than four weeks thereafter, then, subject to subsections (3) to (6), the employee shall not be regarded as having been dismissed by his employer by reason of the ending of his employment under the previous contract.

(3) If, in a case to which subsection (1) applies, the provisions of the contract as renewed, or of the new contract, as to the capacity and place in which the employee is employed, and as to the other terms and conditions of his employment, differ (wholly or in part) from the corresponding provisions of the previous contract, there shall be a trial period in relation to the contract as renewed, or the new contract (whether or not there has been a previous trial under this section).

(6) If during the trial period –

(a) the employee, for whatever reason, terminates the contract, or gives notice to terminate it and the contract is thereafter, in consequence, terminated; or

(b) the employer, for a reason connected with or arising out of the change to the renewed, or new, employment, terminates the contract, or gives notice to terminate it and the contract is thereafter, in consequence, terminated, then, unless the employee's contract of employment is again renewed, or he is again re-engaged under a new contract of employment, in circumstances such that subsection (1) again applies, he shall be treated as having been dismissed.

What legislation supports the mentally handicapped in their attempts to acquire employment and education or training?

Question 9.6

Question 9.7   To what extent can the law both protect the mentally handicapped person and safeguard his freedom in this particular home?

Question 9.8   A number of staff caring for the mentally handicapped have had to make the transition from an institutional to a community setting. How might the law be invoked in these circumstances by both employer and employee?

Can the person working with the mentally handicapped be both friend and professional to his clients?   *Question 9.9*

Activity 9.3

Ask your nearest College of Further Education what facilities are provided for those with learning difficulties.

ANSWERS

Question 9.1

Legislation has involved the local authority in a number of ways with the provision of accommodation for the mentally handicapped.

When a mentally handicapped person has been detained under the Mental Health Act 1983, there is a responsibility on both the health authority and the local social services department to provide aftercare, including domiciliary facilities. The NHS Act 1977 also requires a local authority to cooperate with the health authority 'to advance the health and welfare of the people of England and Wales'.

The Chronically Sick and Disabled Persons Act 1970 places a duty on the local authority to consider the housing needs of the chronically sick or disabled. However this only applies to new housing.

A proportion of housing for the mentally handicapped is provided by the private sector, often voluntary organizations. Under the National Assistance Act 1948, such private homes must be registered and applications for this must be made to the local social services authority. Certain conditions have to be met in order for an application to be approved.

Question 9.2

The first issue is whether Carl has the necessary understanding to be able to consent to treatment. It would be unwise to assume that a patient cannot have this understanding purely on the basis that he is mentally handicapped as there are wide variations in mental impairment. However, there is no doubt that some severely mentally handicapped people are unable to give a valid consent.

A second issue is the role played by the Mental Health Act 1983. Over-ruling of a patient's refusal to give consent can only occur if he is formally detained in hospital and even then there are safeguards as to the nature and duration of the treatment. This legislation cannot be applied in Carl's situation.

Where there is no doubt that the patient is unable to give a valid consent, the doctor might argue that the urgency and necessity of the treatment allows the nurse to proceed with giving the medication and that a failure to treat could even be negligence. This could not apply in this example as Carl may have upset people but he has not harmed them and is not, therefore, a danger to them.

The only other argument to proceed without consent, as seen in T *v*. T 1988 and F *v*. West Berkshire HA 1989, is to consider whether the carrying out of treatment is in the best interests of the patient. A legal action against the nurse or doctor for battery may well not succeed if treatment was given after such consideration and in good faith.

Question 9.3

Outcomes a, b, e, i, j, k and m are all probably involved in the way Pat assesses and plans Carl's care.

Question 9.4

Battery is the application of force to a person against his will. The force need only be slight. There are a number of defences. For example, self-defence is acceptable as long as the force used is reasonable and pro-portionate to the other person's force. Necessity is occasionally a defence but only where the force used is needed to prevent a greater evil. In criminal law, an inability to form the necessary intention will lead to a not guilty finding, but this does not apply in civil law. Finally, consent is a defence.

As none of these apply to John it seems likely that he has committed both the criminal and civil wrong of battery.

The possible outcomes to John are

1. disciplinary action taken by his employer up to or including dismissal;
2. having this incident reported to the UKCC which may take it to the professional conduct committee. The resultant hearing may lead to the removal of his name from the register;
3. the involvement of the police leading to a prosecution and possible criminal conviction;
4. an action in the civil courts brought by Carl's mother on her son's behalf, leading to an award of damages payable by John.

John may have some rights if he is dismissed to appeal against this. The health authority's disciplinary policy is usually in line with the Whitley Council's recommendations which ensure the right of appeal to the nurse manager one level up from the person who has carried out the dismissal. If John has been in employment for a continuous period of two years, he has more extensive rights, including taking his case to an industrial tribunal.

Question 9.5

She would need to write to the appropriate authority responsible for the home. This may not be obvious as responsibility for the care of the mentally handicapped is often shared between the local authority social services department and the health authority, the former being more likely to take the overall control. Even if the home is owned by the health authority, complaints in this setting are outside the Hospital Complaints Procedure Act 1985 but the Health Service Commissioner could possibly become involved.

She could herself complain to the UKCC of the nurse's alleged misconduct which would then have to be investigated.

Question 9.6

There is little legislation that is aimed specifically at the education or employment of the mentally handicapped.

The Education Act 1981 laid a duty on local education authorities to provide 'special educational provision' for children in need. Otherwise local education authorities have a statutory duty to provide full-time education in schools or colleges for all young adults aged 16–19 who request it. It appears that the number of places being offered to mentally handicapped students in Colleges of Further Education has substantially increased over recent years.

The legislation assisting the mentally handicapped person gain employment is mainly the same as for the physically handicapped, i.e. the Disabled Persons Employment Act 1944 and 1958 and the Employment and Training Act 1973. In addition the Mental Health Act 1983 includes a provision for aftercare services by the local authority but these are not specified though could include training facilities.

It should be borne in mind that, as is often the case, the inadequacies of statutory services are often filled by a range of voluntary training and employment services in liaison with the local authority. It seems likely that this relationship will be enhanced on implementation of the Community Care Act 1990.

Question 9.7

The law relating to negligence seems to be the main safety net ensuring the safety of the mentally handicapped person in this kind of community setting. There are staff closely participating in his care and they therefore have a clear duty of care under the law to ensure that no acts or omissions on their part cause resultant harm. As has been demonstrated in several other settings, the law supports the notion of encouraging independence as long as the professional has carefully weighed up both the risks and benefits of such action. This includes a careful assessment of the client's abilities before reducing levels of supervision. The professional must be able to demonstrate that she has acted reasonably.

The issue of safeguards to individual freedoms is more complex. As discussed in question 9.2, there are limitations to what can be done to a patient without his consent. However, there are possible flaws to the argument in F *v.* West Berkshire HA 1989 that the professional can have the power to act in the best interests of the patient who is incapable of giving consent. There is little doubt that professional views vary as to what this means in different cases. At present there is no system of appeal against a medical decision in this situation except to take it through the courts, an unwieldy and expensive business. A complaint to the Community Health Council may serve to raise public awareness of this difficulty.

A final limitation to the freedom of the individual is financial. Financial independence is rarely attained by a mentally handicapped person and reliance on state benefits tends to lead to a fairly minimal standard of living. The relevant legislation tends to discourage the handicapped from working full time in what are usually low paid jobs as this leads to the loss of benefits and a possible reduction in income.

Question 9.8

A number of these issues involve employment legislation. The rate of change in both the health service and the nursing profession has been so rapid over recent years that it is no longer a rare occurrence for contracts to have to be amended or for redundancy to occur. An employment contract must include the names of employer and employee with job title and date of commencement. For the mental handicap nurse, the employer may no longer be the health authority but the local authority. Other details to be included must relate to conditions of employment, although not all the relevant information need be included on the contract as long as the employee is referred to named documents. As these conditions may change it is important that the employee clearly understands what these are as well as what previous entitlements will remain unchanged. As the business of negotiating and agreeing an amended contract is a complex process, the nurse may well decide to involve her union representative.

Changing conditions may lead to the need for new skills and this seems extremely likely in the move from an institutional to a community setting. The employer has a responsibility to provide additional training as does the employee to ask for and accept this. Negligence on the part of the employee in this new setting can thus be avoided and the employing authority protects itself from vicarious liability for the actions of its employees during the course of their duties.

Question 9.9

The legal relevance of this question involves two issues. The first is that the nurse is employed in a certain capacity, i.e. she has a job to do for which she is getting paid. The second is that as a professional she must abide by her Code of Professional Conduct. Breach of this might result in charges of misconduct. Therefore, although the nurse may take on a friendship role within her relationship with her client, her prime responsibility is to act in a professional manner at all times.

RELEVANT STATUTES AND CASES

Chronically Sick and Disabled Persons Act 1970
Community Care Act 1990
Disabled Persons Employment Act 1944 and 1958
Education Act 1981
Employment Protection (Consolidation) Act 1978
Employment and Training Act 1973
Hospital Complaints Procedure Act 1985
Mental Health Act 1983
National Assistance Act 1948
National Health Service Act 1977
National Health Service and Community Care Act 1990
Nurses, Midwives and Health Visitors Act 1979
F. *v.* West Berkshire Health Authority 1989
T. *v* T. 1988

REFERENCES

Bercusson, B. (1976) *The Employment Protection (Consolidation) Act 1978*. Sweet and Maxwell, London.

Boswell, D. and Wingrove, J. (eds) (1974) *The Handicapped Person in the Community*. Oxford University Press and Tavistock Publications.

Department of Health (1990) *The N.H.S. and Community Care Act 1990. A Brief Guide*. Department of Health, London.

Dimond, B. (1990) *Legal Aspects of Nursing*. Prentice Hall, London.

Jones, R. (1985) *Mental Health Act Manual*. Sweet and Maxwell, London.

Pyne, R.H. (1981) *Professional Discipline in Nursing*. Blackwell, Oxford.

Roberts, G. (1978) *Essential Law for Social Workers*. Oyez Publishing Ltd, London.

Taylor, J. (1986) *Mental Handicap. Partnership in the Community?* Office of Health Economics, London.

Topliss, E. and Gould, B. (1981) *A Charter for the Disabled*. Blackwell and Robertson, Oxford.

10 Children's nursing

When Lucy becomes pregnant, she and her husband Greg are thrilled as they have waited eight years for a child. However, tragically, when baby Sarah is born she is found to have a heart defect and requires resuscitation. She survives but the medical and nursing staff soon suspect that Sarah has other defects and a marked hearing impairment is diagnosed.

She makes reasonable progress for the first two years of her life but thereafter her development is slow and her growth retarded compared to other children of the same age. However, in spite of her deafness, she is a mentally alert child who is eager to learn. The general practitioner feels that the only hope for Sarah to lead a relatively normal life is for her to have the cardiac condition corrected by surgery and he asks the cardiac surgeon at the nearest paediatric unit to review her progress. Although the consultant is of the opinion that major cardiac surgery is indicated, he prefers to leave this until Sarah is a little older, seeing her every six months in the meantime.

By the time Sarah is six years old, Lucy and Greg are increasingly worried about her condition. Her mobility is seriously affected, she cannot run as she gets very breathless and her colour is poor. She is often too tired to benefit from the specialist tuition being offered her at her primary school and the slightest infections have Lucy in a state of panic. Sarah's parents become increasingly angry that the hospital consultant is not taking any action but when they push for Sarah's admission they are told that there are children more ill than Sarah and therefore she must wait her turn. Lucy accuses the doctor of putting Sarah to the back of the queue as she has other handicaps.

Read the material below before answering questions 10.1–10.3. You may also find of use the following answers:

Chapter 3 Nos. 2 and 17
Chapter 4 No. 15

Case Studies in Law and Nursing,
Ann P. Young.
Published in 1992 by
Chapman & Hall, London
ISBN 0 412 44130 6.

(A) RE B (A MINOR) (WARDSHIP: MEDICAL TREATMENT) 1981

Baby Alexandra was born with Down's syndrome and an intestinal obstruction. Without surgery (which carried minimal risk) death would occur in a few days. The parents refused to authorize the operation. The doctors informed the local authority who applied to have the child made a ward of court.

The court had to decide whether an operation to relieve an intestinal blockage should be performed on a newborn child suffering from Down's syndrome, who had been made a ward of court. If the operation was not performed the child would die within a matter of days. If it was performed and was successful, the child would probably live for 20 to 30 years – although in a seriously handicapped state. Templeman L.J. said that the decision of the court was 'whether the life of this child is demonstrably going to be so awful that in effect the child must be condemned to die, or whether the life of this child is still so imponderable that it would be wrong for her to be condemned to die'.

He decided that the operation should be performed although he accepted that there might be cases where the life of a child was 'so bound to be full of pain and suffering' that a court might be driven to a different conclusion. The other judge, Dunn L.J., agreed and said that 'here there was no evidence that this child's short life is likely to be an intolerable one'.

Skegg (1984)

(B) R. *v.* LEONARD JOHN HENRY ARTHUR 1981

A baby boy was born with Down's syndrome. The parents did not wish him to survive. Dr Arthur wrote 'Nursing care only' and prescribed dihydrocodeine and water only. The baby died 69 hours after birth.

Dr Arthur was charged with murder, a charge altered to attempted murder as it was impossible to prove that the drug had caused the baby's death and there was no evidence that he had starved to death. The defence established that:

1. the baby suffered severe brain and lung damage;
2. Dr Arthur followed established practice in his management of such an infant;
3. in the first 3 days of life normal babies take little or no sustenance and usually lose weight (which the dead baby had not done).

In Farquharson J.'s direction to the jury he said that it was an important principle in law that 'However serious the case may be, however much the disadvantage of a mongol or indeed any other handicapped child, no doctor has the right to kill it'. There was, he said, no special power, facility or licence to kill children who are handicapped or seriously disadvantaged in any irreversible way.

The motive of alleviating suffering will not provide a legal justification from a doctor who intentionally administers what he knows to be a lethal dose of a drug. Farquharson J. said that it was accepted that the doctor had acted from the highest of motives but directed the jury that 'however noble his motives were, that is irrelevant to the question of your deciding what his intent was.

It may be that somebody faced with an ageing relative who was suffering from an incurably painful disease, from the best motive in the world, decides to put a pillow over the person's head so that he or she dies. That would seem that there was then an intent to kill. The motive of cause would have been the kindest and best'.

Even if a doctor acted in compliance with statements on medical ethics from the BMA, this would not provide a defence if he did any act for the purpose of hastening the death of a patient. Farquharson J. commented that it was customary for a profession to agree on rules of conduct but instructed the jury that 'that does not mean that any profession can set out a code of ethics and say that the law must accept it and take notice of it. Whatever a profession may evolve as a system of standards of ethics cannot stand on its own and cannot survive if it is in conflict with the law'.

Dr Arthur was acquitted.

Brazier (1987), Skegg (1984)

(C) R. *v.* SECRETARY OF STATE FOR SOCIAL SERVICES EX. P. HINCKS AND OTHERS 1979

Orthopaedic patients at a hospital in Birmingham who had waited for treatment for periods longer than was medically advisable, brought an action against the Secretary of State, the regional health authority and the area health authority. They were seeking a declaration that the defendants were in breach of their duty under Section 1 of the National Health Service Act 1977 to promote a comprehensive health service designed to secure improvement in health and the prevention of illness, and under Section 3 to provide accommodation, facilities and services for those purposes.

The judge held that it was not the function of the court to direct Parliament as to what funds to make available to the health service and how to allocate them. The Secretary of State's duty under Section 3 to provide services 'to such extent as he considers necessary', gave him discretion as to the disposition of financial resources. The court could only interfere if the Secretary of State acted so as to frustrate the policy of the Act or as no reasonable minister could have acted. No such breach had been shown in the present case. The court could not grant mandamus or a declaration against area or regional authorities since specific remedies against them were available by Section 85 and Part V of the 1977 Act. Nor if a breach were proved did the Act admit of relief by way of damages. The application was therefore dismissed.

Solicitors Journal, 29 June 1979, 436; in Dimond (1990)

(D) RE WALKER'S APPLICATION 1987

Mrs Walker's baby son required a heart operation and was on the waiting list. A date was fixed for the operation to be performed but was postponed by the Birmingham Health Authority. She applied to the court for a judicial review of the decision of the health authority. The High Court judge refused her application. She appealed to the Court of Appeal who upheld the earlier decision.

The health authority had accepted that the regional health authorities could be subject to judicial review where there was reason to believe that they might be in breach of their public duties. There would always be individuals who believed that treatment was not provided quickly enough, but the financial resources were finite and always would be. The court held that it was not for the court to substitute its own judgement for that of those responsible for the allocation of resources. It would only interfere if there had been a failure to allocate funds in a way which was unreasonable or where there had been breaches of public duties. Mrs Walker's application was refused.

The Times, 26 November 1987; in Dimond (1990)

(E) BULL AND ANOTHER *v.* DEVON AHA 1989

Mrs Bull was carrying twins and went into hospital on Saturday 21 March 1970 when her waters broke prematurely at 33 weeks gestation. Darryl, the first twin, was born at 7.27 pm after a rapid delivery. The second twin, Stuart was delivered 68 minutes later at 8.35 pm.

A senior house officer, who was 25 years old and had been in post three months and a midwifery sister were present. It was accepted that it would have been inappropriate for them to deliver the baby in the circumstances.

There had been an accidental and non-negligent rupture of the second bag of membranes during a vaginal examination by the midwifery sister. The brisk bleeding made delivery of the second twin an urgent necessity. The second twin should have been delivered as soon as reasonably practical after the first, in any event within 20 minutes. The court found that the 68-minute delay was unacceptably long.

Attempts had been made to contact the registrar without success. At 7.55 pm the consultant obstetrician was informed and arrived shortly before 8.25 pm. The consultant carried out the delivery promptly and properly but Stuart subsequently was found to have brain damage.

The plaintiff had established the delay and that it was by 1970 standards unreasonable. The defendants could not prove otherwise and liability was established. Lord Justice Slade, one of the judges in the case, stated: 'This is a case where on the evidence the delays in summoning and securing the attendance of the registrar or consultant were so substantial as to place upon the authority the evidential burden of justifying them if it could, under the *res ipsa loquitur* principle.'

The call system had broken down. Lord Justice Slade also stated that the system was 'precarious' and was 'operating on a knife edge'. Another judge in the case, Lord Justice Dillion, stated that there should have been a staff, 'reasonably sufficient for the foreseeable requirements of the patient'. The delay arising from the hospital's breach of duty was the cause of *intra partum* asphyxia which itself caused Stuart's brain damage.

On 13 November 1989 damages of £750,000 were awarded.

Tingle (1990)

Question 10.1

What is the difference between notification and registration of a birth?

Question 10.2

How may the law become involved when a baby is born with serious handicaps?

Who makes decisions regarding that baby's future?

What does the law have to add to the debate on the use of scarce resources in the National Health Service? *Question 10.3*

Activity 10.1

Find out the longest and shortest waiting lists in your hospital.

Shortly after this, Lucy and Greg separate. Lucy's time and effort have been spent so exclusively on Sarah that the two find that they have drifted apart. In addition, since her birth, Greg has always found it difficult to accept Sarah's disabilities. Lucy then throws herself even more wholeheartedly into trying to get treatment for Sarah. Eventually a surgeon at a specialist hospital agrees to see Sarah and carries out a series of extensive tests on her. His conclusion is that she is a very sick child and the only chance of giving her a reasonable prognosis is a heart transplant.

Lucy writes to Greg to give him this news but he does not reply to her. Instead he telephones the consultant to tell him that he will not give his consent to such an operation. On hearing this Lucy contacts her health visitor, Tom, whom she knows well as he has been involved with the family since Sarah's birth. He in turn contacts the consultant and they meet to discuss the family situation and what action to take. There are a number of options open to them but Tom suggests he tries to find out Greg's objections and talk it through with him.

During this discussion, Greg expresses the opinion that Sarah's quality of life will never be good even if a transplant is successful. Tom manages to clear up some of Greg's misconceptions about transplant surgery and eventually Greg is prepared to allow the doctors to give Sarah a chance of a better future.

Read the material below before answering questions 10.4–10.7. You may also find of use the following answers:

Chapter 1 No. 3
Chapter 6 Nos. 3, 8 and 9

(F) HUMAN TISSUE ACT 1961

Under Section 1(1) of the Human Tissue Act: If any person, either in writing at any time or orally in the presence of two or more witnesses during his last illness, had expressed a request that his body or any specific part of his body be used after his death for therapeutic purposes, or for the purpose of medical education, or research, the person lawfully in possession of his body after his death may, unless he has reason to believe that the request was subsequently withdrawn, authorize the removal from the body of any part or, as the case may be, the specified part, for use in accordance with the request.

The presence of the donor card will count as evidence that the deceased agreed to the use of his body. The card may constitute a general consent or it may be specific. Under this section the person lawfully in charge of the body does not have to carry out reasonable enquiries to ascertain if the deceased had changed his mind. All that is necessary is that he has no reason to believe that the request was withdrawn.

Under Section 1(2) of the Human Tissue Act the person lawfully in charge of the body of a deceased person may authorize the removal of any part from the body for use for the said purposes (therapeutic, or medical education, or research) if having made such reasonable enquiry as may be practicable, he has no reason to believe: (a) that the deceased had expressed an objection to his body being so dealt with after his death, and had not withdrawn it; or (b) that the surviving spouse or any surviving relative of the deceased objects to the body being so dealt with.

(G) GILLICK v. WEST NORFOLK AND WISBECH AHA AND THE DHSS 1985

Mrs Gillick questioned the lawfulness of a DHSS circular HN(80)46 which was a revised version of part of a comprehensive *Memorandum of Guidance* on family planning services issued to health authorities in May 1974 under cover of circular HSC(IS)32. The circular stated that in certain circumstances a doctor could lawfully prescribe contraception for a girl under 16 without the consent of the parents. Mrs Gillick wrote to the acting administrator formally forbidding any medical staff employed by the Norfolk AHA to give 'any contraceptive or abortion or treatment whatever to my...daughters whilst they are under 16 years without my consent'. The administrator replied that the treatment prescribed by a doctor is a matter for the doctor's clinical judgement, taking into account all the factors of the case. Mrs Gillick, who had five daughters, then brought an action against the AHA and the DHSS seeking a declaration that the notice gave advice which was unlawful and wrong and which did or might adversely affect the welfare of her children, her right as a parent and her ability properly to discharge her duties as a parent. She sought a declaration that no doctor or other professional person employed by the health authority might give any contraceptive or abortion advice or treatment to any of her children below the age of 16 without her prior knowledge and consent.

She failed before the High Court judge, succeeded in her appeal before the Court of Appeal and the DHSS and Health Authority appealed to the House of Lords. The Lords decided by a majority of 3 to 2 against Mrs Gillick. The majority held that in exceptional circumstances a doctor could provide contraceptive advice and treatment to a girl under 16 without the parent's consent. The circular was therefore upheld.

Lord Fraser stated the exceptional circumstances as follows:

1. the girl would, although under 16, understand the doctor's advice;
2. he could not persuade her to inform her parents or allow him to inform the parents that she was seeking contraceptive advice;
3. she was very likely to have sexual intercourse with or without contraceptive treatment;
4. unless she received contraceptive advice or treatment her physical or mental health or both were likely to suffer and;
5. her best interests required him to give her contraceptive advice, treatment or both without parental consent.

Lord Soarman stated that

1. parental rights are derived from parental duties and these duties are only needed until the child is sufficiently capable of making his own decisions. Therefore, parental rights are not absolute;
2. the common law had never regarded the child's consent as complete nullity.

(H) FAMILY LAW REFORM ACT 1969

Section 8

The consent of a minor who has attained the age of 16 years to any surgical, medical or dental treatment, which in the absence of consent would constitute a trespass to his person will be as effective as it would be if he were of full age: and where a minor has by virtue of this section given an effective consent to any treatment, it shall not be necessary to obtain any consent for it from his parent or guardian.

(I) CHILDREN ACT 1989

Part I

The child's welfare must be the paramount consideration of the court and the court must consider specific circumstances included in the welfare checklist when deciding the child's future.

This checklist includes the 'ascertainable wishes and feelings of the child concerned', his needs, the likely effect of any change of circumstances, any relevant characteristics, any harm or risk of harm, how capable are the parents.

The Act defines parental responsibility, replacing the former concept of parental rights.

There is a duty for local authorities to find out and consider the views of children and their parents.

Part II

This lays down the orders with respect to children in family proceedings.

1. Contact order.
2. Residence order.
3. Specific issue order.
4. Prohibited steps order.

Part III

This draws together local authorities' principal functions in providing support for children and families. It imposes a general duty on local authorities to 'safeguard and promote the welfare of children within their area who are in need'. It goes on to define when a child is in need.

Part IV

A court order giving parental responsibility to the local authority will only be made if the order will contribute positively to the child's welfare. Care and supervision orders are available.

Part V

This includes several orders for the protection of children.

1. Child Assessment Order.
2. Emergency Protection Order (replacing the previous Place of Safety Order).

Part VI

This covers local authority provided, assisted and controlled homes.

Part VII

This covers voluntary homes and organizations.

Part VIII

This provides for the registration and regulation of private children's homes, including foster carers.

Part IX

This controls private fostering arrangements.

Part X

This part defines and provides for the registration of child minders.

Adapted from Leenders (1990)

What legal controls are there over organ donation?
Who gives consent for an organ to be removed from a body?

Question 10.4

Question 10.5

What rights and responsibilities do parents have over their children in relation to medical treatment?
What degree of choice might a child have with regard to medical treatment?

Question 10.6

In what ways may parental responsibilities be removed?
How are parental rights and responsibilities complicated when parents are separated or divorced?

What information issues concerning Sarah's treatment are illustrated at this point in the case study?
Do they have a legal component?

Activity 10.2
Look at the wording on a donor card.

The wait for a suitable donor lasts four months until a 10-year-old child is knocked off her bicycle and sustains serious head injuries. Although she is put on a life support system, she is pronounced dead 48 hours later. Fortunately for Sarah, the parents of this child have already let it be known that they wish their daughter's organs to be used to save another person's life. Sarah is admitted to hospital and prepared for surgery. At the same time, the ventilator is turned off and a team remove the donor heart.

Surgery goes smoothly but while the operation is being completed Sarah's blood pressure plummets. In spite of efforts to restore her circulation, she dies in theatre.

Lucy seems to accept that everything possible was done for her child but Greg is sure that there has been some fault on the part of the doctors and nurses. He asks for information as to what went wrong but receives such a bland reply that he writes again, threatening to sue. However, on taking legal advice, he manages to get access to Sarah's medical and nursing notes and eventually has to accept that there is no evidence of negligence. Sarah's death was unavoidable.

Read the material below before answering questions 10.8–10.10. In addition you may find of use the following answers:

Chapter 2 No. 3
Chapter 6 Nos. 10 and 16

Material in Chapter 7 is also relevant.

(J) R. *v.* MALCHEREK 1981

The victim of assault was maintained on a ventilator until the doctors were of the opinion that brain death had occurred. The assailants contended that the cause of death was the termination of artifical ventilation. The original trial accepted that the victim was dead after brain death even if the heart still beats. The Appeal Court argued a different point; Lord Lane stated, 'There is no evidence in the present case that at the time of conventional death, after the life support machinery was disconnected, the original wound or injury was other than a continuing, operating and indeed substantial cause of the death of the victim'.

Skegg (1984)

(K) ROE *v.* MINISTER OF HEALTH 1954

During the course of an operation, the plaintiff was paralyzed by anaesthetic which had become contaminated by disinfectant. The anaesthetic had been kept in glass ampoules which were stored in the disinfectant and became contaminated by seepage through invisible cracks in the glass. At the time of the accident in 1947 this risk was not known. The Court of Appeal held that the hospital authorities were not liable because the danger was not reasonably foreseeable. The court 'must not look at the 1947 accident with 1954 spectacles' opined Denning L.I. but it would have been negligent to adopt the same practice in 1954.

Tyas (1989)

In situations of brain stem death, who decides when the life support   *Question 10.8*
systems are to be discontinued?

In the operating theatre, what situations of potential negligence can   *Question 10.9*
arise in which the nurse may have played a part?

Question 10.10   How can Greg legally get access to information about Sarah's treatment and death?
What practical limitations might he find if he decided to sue the
hospital for negligence?

Activity 10.3
When you visit the operating theatre, observe how nurses attempt to
reduce the risk of accidents.

ANSWERS

Question 10.1

Notification of a birth must be done within 36 hours to the local medical officer of health by the person in attendance on the woman during childbirth. This will often be the midwife.

Every birth must also be registered within 6 weeks to the District Registrar of Births, Marriages and Deaths. This is usually done by the parents but if this is not possible, any other qualified informant has a duty to do so.

Question 10.2

There have been a number of instances where the parents have rejected their handicapped baby. The local authority must then use a care and supervision order under the Children Act 1989. The preconditions for this are that the child is suffering or is likely to suffer significant harm because of a lack of reasonable parental care. In these circumstances the local authority then has the responsibility of making decisions regarding the child's future. As a safety net, if there is potential conflict concerning the local authority's decisions, the High Court can intervene. For example, baby Alexandra (Re B (A Minor) (Wardship: Medical Treatment) 1981) was put into the care of the local authority after the doctors brought the situation to its attention and the baby was then made a ward of court for a decision on a potentially controversial issue.

Parents may go a stage further than rejection and actively seek to prevent any treatment for the newborn baby. Baby Alexandra's parents refused consent for life saving surgery. The parents of a baby boy also with Down's syndrome and born in 1981, made it clear to Dr Arthur that they did not wish the baby to survive. However the law does not support the parents' wishes over and above any other factors and therefore the law accepts that the decision may be taken from them. In R. *v.* Arthur 1981, it was Dr Arthur who took the decision as to how to treat the baby rather than taking the case to the local authority.

Although it is likely that in similar circumstances it is often the paediatrician or obstetrician who takes on the responsibility for deciding how to treat the newborn handicapped child, the legal outcome for Dr Arthur in deciding to sedate and withhold nutrition from the baby was a prosecution for murder, later changed to attempted murder. For a number of reasons he was acquitted. Where there is difficulty in deciding what is in the best interests of the baby in relation to his quality of life it does seem wiser to involve the local authority and potentially the courts.

Question 10.3

The National Health Service Act 1977 allows discretion as to the extent of service provision within the wider responsibility of promoting a comprehensive health service. It is therefore extremely difficult to argue the improper use of resources under this statute.

In Re Walker's Application 1987, Mrs Walker failed to gain a judicial review of the health authority's decision over the use of resources. However, although the court stated that it was not for the court to substitute its own judgement for that of those responsible, it did not rule out a role for the court in future disputes if the allocation of funds was unreasonable or in breach of public duties.

There is no doubt that health authority managers are in a predicament. Resources will always be less than ideal and therefore decisions have to be made on financial and ethical grounds rather than legal ones. In addition, the temptation to accept more patients than the resources can support has to be resisted. Any resultant harm, for example because of a lack of trained staff and proper equipment, could be negligence, as illustrated in the Bull case.

Question 10.4

The law is somewhat complex in this area. The Human Tissue Act 1961 is the main legislation stating that parts of the human body can be removed after death 'for therapeutic purposes or for purposes of medical education and research'. The deceased person may or may not have made his wishes known as to the use of his body for organ donation before his death. The existence of a donor card will help to provide evidence of the deceased person's wishes. However, in either case authorization has to be given by the person lawfully in possession of the body and this is where legal difficulties may arise.

The Anatomy Act 1984 supports the view that the hospital authority is legally in possession (assuming the person died in hospital) until the body is claimed and during this time certain designated persons can remove parts of the body for therapeutic purposes. However possession rights can be claimed by a number of other people and under common law the next of kin are entitled to possession of the body in the same condition as when death occurred, and the right to dispose of the body is usually seen to belong to the close relatives. In addition, the coroner may have possession rights for a period of time.

Who gives consent for organ removal depends to a large extent on the interpretation of the phrase 'after making reasonable enquiry' (Section 1(2) of the Human Tissue Act). Because of the common law situation, the consent of the relatives is gained if at all possible. However, as decisions often have to be made rapidly, the hospital authority may interpret 'reasonable enquiry' in a less stringent manner than the relatives might wish for. Whatever the situation, it is clear that the existence of a donor card cannot automatically give consent to the removal of organs.

Question 10.5

Parental responsibility includes all the rights, powers, authority and duties of parents in relation to a child and his property (Section 3(1) of the Children Act 1989). The subsuming of parental rights under responsibility more accurately reflects that the true nature of these rights is limited to how parents may carry out their duties.

Thus parents have a duty to ensure that the child receives proper medical attention until the child is old enough to make decisions for himself. Under the Family Law Reform Act 1969 this is when the child reaches the age of 16 years. However, the law has never considered that under this age, parental rights are absolute and in some circumstances if the child has sufficient understanding and maturity, his consent will be acceptable. This is particularly clear in an emergency but now can apply on the issue of contraception and medical treatment (Gillick *v.* West Norfolk and Wisbech AHA and the DHSS 1985).

Question 10.6

A child must be protected from the harm which can arise from failures or abuse within the family. The Children Act 1989 authorizes a number of interventions which give the courts discretion to implement a variety of orders.

1. Care and Supervision Orders are used if a child is suffering or likely to suffer significant harm because of a lack of reasonable parental care.
2. Interim Care and Supervision Orders are used if the court concludes there are reasonable grounds for believing the above.
3. Emergency Protection Orders are used if there is reasonable cause to believe that the child is likely to suffer significant harm unless he is removed to another place.
4. Child Assessment Orders can be used where there is no emergency but the likelihood of significant harm needs to be explored in situations where parents are uncooperative.

Where parents have been married at or after the time of the child's conception, parental responsibilities are always shared and this does not alter after separation or divorce. A difficulty could potentially arise where each parent is exercising his or her responsibility independently (as in Sarah's case). Under the Children Act 1989 there is no duty imposed on one parent to consult with the other nor is there a right of veto of one parent against the action of the other. It therefore seems to be acceptable for the doctor or nurse to accept the consent of the parent who is caring for the child as it is she who needs to be able to respond to circumstances as they arise, i.e. Lucy's consent would be adequate.

Question 10.7

1. The mother informs her estranged husband of their child's planned treatment. Legally she does not have to do so and a parent would need to ask the court to make an order requiring the other parent to keep him/her informed before a particular step is taken.

2. The health visitor shares information about the family with the consultant. There are no legal components to this action although ethically the health visitor should have asked Lucy's permission to do so.
3. The consultant and the health visitor make a decision to include the father in further discussion. Legally the consent of the father is not needed as he cannot prevent treatment to which the other parent has agreed. Therefore this decision has no legal significance.
4. The health visitor imparts information of a medical nature to the father that is usually the responsibility of the doctor. If the information had been wrong and this led to harm, then the health visitor might have been negligent. However, it is difficult to envisage how harm might occur in these particular circumstances.

Question 10.8

Medical staff have the responsibility of deciding when to discontinue life support systems after brain stem death has occurred. Usually the decision is seen as being made by the medical team rather than by one doctor, the burden of such responsibility being better shared. It is not the responsibility of the relatives and it may be the nurse who has to explain to them that death has in fact occurred before the machine is turned off.

The precise time of the discontinuation of life support may be influenced by a number of factors. If an organ is to be removed for donation, this may be delayed until a potential recipient is under preparation. The final act may also be postponed if relatives are so distressed that they are unable to accept reality.

Question 10.9

1. An operation may be carried out on the wrong patient. The nurse receiving the patient from the ward has a responsibility to check the identity of the patient.
2. An operation may be carried out on the wrong part of the body, for example the left leg instead of the right leg. A nurse must never be involved in marking the patient's body prior to surgery. The theatre nurse must ensure that the correct medical notes are received with the patient.
3. Swabs or instruments may be left inside a patient at the end of the operation. The theatre nurses have strict responsibilities in relation to counting swabs and instruments both prior to their use and on removal from the patient. A failure to do so with resultant harm will always be negligence.
4. Spillage of lotions or other fluids on the floor of the operating theatre could lead to staff slipping with possible harm to the patient. Nurses have a responsibility to maintain a safe environment.
5. Careless handling of a patient while under anaesthetic could be

negligence. The nurse may be involved here along with other theatre personnel.

Question 10.10

Once a legal action has been started, the court can order the release of medical and nursing documentation to the plaintiff. It is possible to request access to medical notes under the Access to Health Records Act 1990. However, the doctor can block this if he considers that it would be harmful to the patient's physical or mental health (not applicable in this situation). There is a similar right under the Data Protection Act 1984 for information held on computer.

As Sarah's death occurred during the operative period, the coroner would have to be informed. Greg would probably have gained a great deal of information from the coroner's hearing as well as being able to ask questions of the witnesses.

There are a number of practical difficulties in suing for negligence. The first consideration may well be financial. Legal aid is only available to those on very limited incomes and legal costs are heavy. If the case were lost by Greg he may in addition have to pay the legal costs of the defence.

For a successful action for negligence, there must be a breach of duty and resultant harm. Even if a failure in that duty could be found, resultant harm may be difficult to prove. In such major and relatively new surgery, carried out on a sick individual, the risks are high. Death may well have been unavoidable.

RELEVANT STATUTES AND CASES

Access to Health Records Act 1990
Anatomy Act 1984
Children Act 1989
Data Protection Act 1984
Family Law Reform Act 1969
Human Tissue Act 1961
National Health Service Act 1977
Bull and Another *v.* Devon AHA 1989
Gillick *v.* West Norfolk and Wisbech AHA and the DHSS 1985
Re B (A Minor) (Wardship: Medical Treatment) 1981
Re Walker's Application 1987
R. *v.* Arthur 1981
R. *v.* Malcherek 1981
R. *v.* Secretary of State for Social Services 1979
Roe *v.* Minister of Health 1954

REFERENCES

Brazier, M. (1987) *Medicine, Patients and the Law*. Penguin, Harmondsworth, Middlesex.

Department of Health (1989) *An Introduction to the Children Act 1989.* HMSO, London.

Dimond, B. (1990) *Legal Aspects of Nursing.* Prentice Hall, London.

Leenders, F. (1990) Children first. *Community Outlook*, July 1990, pp. 4–6.

Medical Defence Union and Royal College of Nursing (1978) *Safeguards against Failure to Remove Swabs and Instruments from Patients.* MDU, London.

Medical Defence Union and Royal College of Nursing (1983) *Safeguards against Wrong Operations.* MDU, London.

Medical Defence Union, Royal College of Nursing, National Association of Theatre Nurses (1988) *Theatre Safeguards* (revised). MDU, London.

Skegg, P.D.G. (1984) *Law, Ethics and Medicine.* Oxford University Press, Oxford.

Tingle, J. (1990) The important case of Bull. *Nursing Standard*, **37**(4), 54–5.

Tyas, J.G.M. (1989) *Law of Torts*, 5th edn. M and E Handbooks, McDonald and Evans Ltd., Plymouth.

PART THREE

Preparation for Registration –

Level 3

Read the following case study and see how many points you can identify that have legal implications for the nurse. I suggest you mark the relevant line in the margin. You should note at least 16 points but may find as many as 24 points.

Brenda has just qualified and is taking up a staff nurse post on an orthopaedic ward. This was not her first choice of job as she has not had experience of orthopaedic nursing since a short placement early in her training. However, she now feels quite enthusiastic about the post and starts her first shift at 07.30 on a Monday morning.

Monday is a busy day as there is a full theatre list as well as a number of patients requiring a great deal of nursing care. Brenda is asked to supervise a first year student nurse for the morning. She divides the work between the two of them. She delegates the preparation of one patient for theatre to the student while she goes to prepare a second patient. However, the student says she is unsure what to do so Brenda quickly runs over the procedure. When the premedication of omnopon and scopolamine is due for the first patient, she takes the student with her to the C.D. cupboard and checks the drug with her. They then give the drug and sign the C.D. book. Forty minutes later the porter arrives for the patient and Brenda takes the medical notes and X-rays with her and accompanies the patient to the operating theatre where she hands over to the theatre nurse.

By lunchtime, the ward has become even busier with several patients back from theatre, an emergency admission from the Accident and Emergency Department on his way up to the ward and some relatives wanting to speak to Brenda. In addition, the lunch trolley has arrived and some prelunch drugs still have to be given. Another staff nurse notices that Brenda is looking harassed and comes to help her. Eventually the urgent tasks are dealt with and lunches are served. Several patients complain that their food is cold and Brenda apologizes.

The newly admitted patient is seen by the doctor who orders skin traction and Brenda sets this up with the student before they go to have their own lunch. On returning from lunch, Brenda is called into

Case Studies in Law and Nursing,
Ann P. Young.
Published in 1992 by
Chapman & Hall, London
ISBN 0 412 44130 6.

the office by the ward sister who has just come on duty. She tells Brenda that she set up the skin traction wrongly as she failed to tilt the end of the bed, and that such mistakes are not acceptable. The sister tells Brenda that the mistake has been rectified and hopefully no harm has been done.

Brenda then hands over her patients to a nurse on the late shift and she and the student complete the nursing records of the morning's care. At 14.30 most of the nursing staff congregate for a teaching session to revise lifting techniques. The session is run by a physiotherapist and a nurse who has recently attended an updating session in the School of Nursing.

The early part of the evening is reasonably quiet but at 18.30 one of the trained nurses has to go off duty as she has just had a message that her husband has been injured in a car accident. This leaves the ward short-staffed. The ward sister feels that they can manage until an elderly patient becomes confused and falls out of bed and the blood pressure of one of the postoperative patients drops. The sister then bleeps the nursing officer to ask for help but the nursing officer says that there is no other nurse that she can send.

The house officer has to be called several times during the next two hours and is feeling hard-pressed herself. While she is writing up the medical notes she asks a staff nurse to prepare a drug for intravenous administration. This she checks with the nurse and then asks her to go and give it. The nurse explains to the doctor that she is not qualified to do this.

At the end of the late shift the sister sends the day staff off duty on time but she herself stays on the ward for an extra hour with the night staff. Eventually she goes off duty once she feels that it is safe to do so.

ANSWERS

Line 1
Qualification involves the completion of a training approved by the National Board. The nurse must then apply to be placed on the relevant part of the Register as required by the UKCC.
(See Question 9.4).

Line 1
Brenda would have agreed an employment contract for this post.
(See Chapter 12).

Line 8
Supervision of students is probably included in Brenda's job description. There are also legal implications to the level of supervision required: the less experienced the person giving care, the greater the duty on the trained nurse to supervise her by working closely with her.
(See Question 5.8).

Line 9

Brenda is potentially negligent in the way she delegates care to the student. If harm resulted from some failure of the student to give proper care, Brenda could be sued for negligent delegation. She does then partially remedy this failure by running over the procedure.
(See Question 3.9).

Line 11

Inexperience is no excuse for negligent care. The student very rightly realizes her limitations and seeks to remedy the situation.
(See Question 4.14).

Line 14, 15

Certain drugs, e.g. omnopon, are controlled by the Misuse of Drugs Act 1971 which lays down certain requirements regarding storage and recording of these drugs. In addition local hospital policy regarding checking and administration of drugs must be followed.
(See Question 5.9).

Line 17

The ward nurse has a duty to identify the patient to the theatre nurse as well as handing over the correct medical notes.
(See Question 10.9).

Line 23

The nursing staff have a legal duty to give treatment prescribed by a doctor, unless the order is clearly unreasonable.
(See Question 7.2).

Line 24

Nurses are tempted to try and cope whatever the odds. The nurse should bear in mind that it is far preferable to ask for help and avoid harm to her patients.
(See Question 3.3).

Line 24

Priorities have to be organized. The law on negligence is helpful here as it supports the notion of safe care and safety needs are a good basis for deciding priorities.
(See Question 2.4).

Line 26

Most hospitals have a complaints policy in line with the requirements of the Hospital Complaints Procedure Act 1985. However, it is always important to try to resolve complaints at an early stage to prevent them from escalating unnecessarily.
(See Question 3.18).

Line 32

Brenda's mistake could be classed as misconduct although of a fairly minor kind. Thus the sister is justified in disciplining her.
(See Question 2.10).

Line 33

For negligence, harm must result, so although Brenda failed in her duty of care to the patient, she is not legally negligent.
(See Question 5.4).

Line 35

When handing over to another nurse, it is important to ensure that no information is omitted that could lead to negligence. Any instructions or changes in the patient's condition must be stated clearly.
(See Questions 3.6 and 5.13)

Line 36

Nursing records are potential legal documents and must be completed carefully and accurately and then signed. Brenda must remember that she is still supervising the student and therefore ensure that any records that the student completes are checked.
(See Questions 2.11 and 2.12).

Line 37

Instruction in proper lifting techniques is an important managerial function under the Health and Safety at Work (etc.) Act 1974. Employees have a duty to cooperate in any training.
(See Questions 2.8 and 7.3).

Line 39

The nurse has a duty to update knowledge. A failure to do so could be negligence.
(See Question 5.6).

Line 42

Conditions of service usually allow paid special leave for family bereavement or serious illness.

Line 45

There will be a question as to whether there is negligence in this situation. The law will always look at what is reasonable in specific circumstances. On the one hand, if it was known that there was a likelihood of the patient getting confused, steps should have been taken to safeguard the patient. On the other hand, if this eventuality was difficult to predict and bearing in mind the staffing levels and the dependency of other patients at that time, then the duty of care towards the elderly patient may have been adequate. Documentation of *all* relevant details is vital.
(See Question 2.4).

Line 46

The fact that this patient's blood pressure falls is likely to be due to the trauma of the operation. However, a failure by the nursing staff to report this change could be evidence of negligence.
(See Question 6.16).

Line 47, 48

The sister is acting correctly in reporting her concern about staffing levels on the ward. It is important that the sister records her action and the nursing officer's response. If harm did result due to a failure of the ward staff to give safe care to all the patients, it is likely that any negligence would have been passed to the nursing officer due to her failure to provide a safe system. Of course, the nursing officer may well have a major problem in ensuring adequate staff cover. Sickness levels and an inadequate budget can make the provision of safe care difficult. She in turn has a duty to plan efficiently (and assist her subordinate to do so as well) and argue effectively with her own manager in order to improve the situation.
(See Questions 4.15 and 10.3).

Line 52

When doctor and nurse share the checking of medication, the duty to ensure that this is done properly is also shared. Thus any mistake that harms the patient would be negligence on the part of them both. The nurse cannot argue as an excuse that she followed the doctor's instructions when the drug being checked is one of which she should have knowledge.
(See Question 2.9).

Line 53

The nurse is only allowed to take on responsibilities that are normally undertaken by a doctor under certain controlled conditions (see the DHSS circular reproduced on pp. 186–188). A decision by the nurse to proceed without these controls would increase the risk of harm to the patient as well as placing herself outside of the covering (vicarious) liability of the hospital employer for her acts. The giving of intravenous drugs is clearly an extension to the nurse's normal role but many other extensions are met, particularly in specialist units or departments, for example suturing, applying plaster of paris, administering ventricular defibrillation and prescribing certain drugs.
(See Question 6.15).

Line 57

The ward sister is contracted to work a stated number of hours. If she left the ward before ensuring the safety of her patients she may feel morally at fault but at present the way nursing is organized does mean that she can safely hand over responsibility to someone else.
(See Chapter 12).

HEALTH CIRCULAR   HC(77)22

DEPARTMENT OF HEALTH AND SOCIAL SECURITY

June 1977

THE EXTENDING ROLE OF THE CLINICAL NURSE –
LEGAL IMPLICATIONS & TRAINING REQUIREMENTS

SUMMARY

In recent years nurses in both primary and specialist health care have become increasingly involved in tasks, procedures and decision making which have in the past been a medical responsibility. This trend is the result of a number of factors including the increasing complexity of treatment and the growth in the specialist expertise of the nurse. The trend has caused some uncertainty about legal implications and training requirements among both professions and employing authorities, and the Department has been urged to issue guidance on the matter. CMO/CNO letter dated 30 June (copy enclosed) explains the professional background.

BACKGROUND

1.1   *The Committee on Nursing (Briggs Report)*

The Committee on Nursing under the Chairmanship of Professor Asa Briggs had as its terms of reference:

'To review the role of the nurse and the midwife in the hospital and the community and the education and training required for that role, so that the best use is made of available manpower to meet present needs and the needs of an integrated health service'.

In its report (published October 1972) the Committee considered the question of overlapping functions. It emphasised the essential differences between the caring role of nurses and the diagnostic and curative functions of doctors. It recognised that some of the differences in function were becoming less distinguishable and emphasised the need for closer co-operation between the two professions in the best interests of the patient.

In considering legal aspects of the relative responsibilities of doctors and nurses the Committee concluded that though there were no apparent legal objections to continuing the existing practice of dividing work between the professions nurses should be required to undertake only those duties for which they had been educated and trained.

1.2   *The Joint Working Party*

In February 1974, an informal discussion was held between officers of the Department and representatives of the major medical and nursing professional organisations at which it was confirmed that the matters raised in the discussion paper required urgent consideration and that guidance was needed. It was agreed that the professional organisations would nominate representatives to participate, together with officers of the Department in a joint working party with the following terms of reference:

'to identify areas of clinical practice in which the role of nurses (except midwives and those whose service is not the responsibility of the Department) is extending in relation to that of doctors, taking into account the legal, ethical and training implications, with a view to establishing whether guidance to employing authorities and the professions is required'.

The joint working party undertook a small fact finding survey of what tasks nurses were currently undertaking which appeared to represent an extension of the nurse's traditional role. The recommendations in this note of guidance are based upon the discussions with professional organisations who were consulted about the Report.

THE ROLE OF THE NURSE

2.1 *The Basic Role*

The International Council of Nurses' definition of a nurse states that a nurse is a person who has completed a programme of basic nursing education and is qualified and authorised in her/his country to practise nursing which involves the promotion of health, the prevention of illness, the care of the sick and rehabilitation. Basic nursing education is a planned educational programme which provides a broad and sound foundation for the practice of nursing and for post basic education.

No profession whose functions are as diverse as nursing can maintain or improve standards of health care and be flexible enough to meet continually changing demands unless continuous attention is given to education and to the planning and evaluation of experimental studies designed to improve nursing practices.

However, whatever changes may occur at the perimeter of the nurse's professional role, caring for people remains the essence of the exercise of her profession.

2.2 *The Extending Role*

The role of the nurse is continually developing as changes in practice and training add new functions to her normal range of duties. Over and above this, however, the clinical nursing role in relation to that of the doctor may be extended in two ways, viz. by delegation by the doctor and in response to emergency. Where delegation occurs, the doctor remains responsible for his patient and for the overall management of treatment, and the nurse is responsible for carrying out delegated tasks competently. A case in point is the involvement of nurses in immunisation procedures which was the subject of Health Circular (76)26, issued in May 1976.

LEGAL IMPLICATIONS

3. In an action for damages, a nurse may be held legally liable if it can be shown either that she has failed to exercise the skills properly expected of her, or that she has undertaken tasks she was not competent to perform. The doctor may be held to be guilty of negligent delegation if it can be shown that he conferred authority on a nurse to perform a task which was either outside the scope of the duties she was normally expected to perform, or for which she had no special qualification. Work which has hitherto been carried out by doctors ought therefore to be delegated to nurses only when: –

    a.   The nurse has been specifically and adequately trained for the performance of the new task and she agrees to undertake it;
    b.   this training has been recognised as satisfactory by the employing Authority;
    c.   the new task has been recognised by the professions and by the employing authority as a task which may be properly delegated to a nurse;
    d.   the delegating doctor has been assured of the competence of the individual nurse concerned.

ACTION

In the interests of providing an effective service to meet the needs of patients within available resources, Health Authorities are asked to review areas where delegation to nurses is desirable. In order to be successful and safe such delegation should be in the context of a clearly defined policy based on prior local discussion and agreement between those responsible for providing nursing and medical services, and it should be made known in writing to all staff who are likely to be involved. In order to safeguard the Health Authorities' liability for the actions of the staff in their employ, the policy should specify: –

a.   what tasks may be delegated,
b.   what qualifications and training are necessary before a nurse may accept particular delegated tasks, and
c.   what safeguards must accompany the delegation of particular tasks in order that the safety of the patient is not jeopardised.

RELEVANT STATUTES AND CASES

Health and Safety at Work (etc.) Act 1974
Hospital Complaints Procedure Act 1985
Misuse of Drugs Act 1971
Nurses, Midwives and Health Visitors Act 1979
Barnett *v.* Chelsea and Kensington H.M.C. 1969
Hunter *v.* Hanley 1955
Wilsher *v.* Essex Area Health Authority 1988

REFERENCES

Brazier, M. (1987) *Medicine, Patients and the Law*, Penguin, Harmondsworth, Middlesex.

Carson, D. and Montgomery, J. (1989) *Nursing and the Law.* Macmillan, Basingstoke, Hampshire.

DHSS (1977) *The Extending Role of the Clinical Nurse.* HC(77)22. DHSS, London.

Health and Safety Commission (1988) *Handling Loads at Work. Proposals for Regulations and Guidance.* Health and Safety Executive, London.

Marsh, G. (1984) The Ombudsman functions and jurisdiction. *Nursing Times*, **80**, 47.

Medical Defence Union, Royal College of Nursing (1983) *Safeguards Against Wrong Operations.* Medical Defence Union, London.

Medical Defence Union, Royal College of Nursing, National Association of Theatre Nurses (1986) *Theatre Safeguards.* Medical Defence Union, London.

Senior, O.E. (1979) *Dependency and Establishments.* Royal College of Nursing, London.

Senior, O.E. (1988) Manpower planning objectives and information systems, in D. Hudson (ed.) *Recent Advances in Nursing: Nursing Administration.* Churchill Livingstone, London.

Tingle, J.H. (1989) Extending capability. *Nursing Standard*, **4**(6), 32.

Young, A.P. (1991) *Law and Professional Conduct in Nursing.* Scutari, London.

Becoming an employee   12

Read the following case study and identify the points that have legal implications, marking the relevant line in the margin. You should identify at least 10 points but may find as many as 15.

When Roger qualifies as a children's nurse, he is undecided as to the field in which he wants to specialise. He decides that he will work as an agency nurse for a while as this will take him into a number of different environments and give him a mixture of experiences.

His first assignment is to a children's unit in a private hospital. He is impressed by the appearance of the unit and the overall efficiency of the staff, but he is irritated by the fact that when there is no other staff nurse on duty an enrolled nurse is put in charge over him. He also finds that he is not allowed to take on some of the responsibilities that he was used to during the latter part of his training. However, these restrictions seem to apply to all nursing staff so he does not feel singled out. Another difference from his training that he notices is the appearance on the unit of several 'reps' from various companies supplying equipment and drugs. These reps seem generous in giving pens, diaries and information booklets to the nurses and even laying on occasional study days on specific nursing issues.

Although there are a number of things he enjoys about working in a private hospital, he cannot help but be conscious of the legal differences in the relationship between the staff and the patients, or in this case, their parents. The importance of careful detailing of costs and the very business-like manner of management are new to Roger although he appreciates that such an approach is being implemented in the National Health Service. However, he has enjoyed nursing children with neurological disorders (the speciality of this particular unit), so decides to look for a permanent job in this area, but in the NHS.

An advertisement in a nursing journal catches his attention:

RGN/RSCN – GRADES E and F.

Are you a motivated, enthusiastic paediatric nurse who would like to come and work in our new unit? If so, you can hope to

Case Studies in Law and Nursing,
Ann P. Young.
Published in 1992 by
Chapman & Hall, London
ISBN 0 412 44130 6.

develop your management skills and gain specialist paediatric clinical experience.

We have vacancies on our 28 bedded ward which specialises in neurology, haematology and, most recently, bone marrow transplantation. We also admit children from the Accident and Emergency Department.

We have a friendly progressive unit and we are totally committed to family centred care. There is also opportunity for professional development.

If interested, please contact . . . .

WE ARE AN EQUAL OPPORTUNITIES EMPLOYER.

Roger fills in an application form and is asked to attend for interview. This is not as much of an ordeal as he feared although he is surprised to be asked if he has any criminal convictions. He then has to have a medical examination in the Occupational Health Department. This provokes considerable anxiety in Roger as he is diabetic and has met some difficulties in the past in relation to employment because of this. However, he is reassured that the hospital does not rule out prospective employees because of diabetes as long as they are medically fit.

Roger is offered a staff nurse post at Grade E which he accepts. He starts work and one month later receives his contract which he duly signs. The contract states pay, hours, period of notice and grounds for dismissal as well as referring the employee to other named sources for further information on conditions of service.

He settles into the job quickly, enjoying the work and getting on well with his colleagues. Unfortunately after about one month he picks up a throat infection and has to go off sick. This destabilizes his diabetes so he is off for several weeks and he has several more periods of sickness over the next three months. His manager refers him to the Occupational Health Department for an opinion as to his health and he is seen formally by his manager under the hospital's sickness policy. By this time Roger is very worried that he will be dismissed from his job. However, with ongoing medical supervision and support from his manager, Roger's health improves and he is able to return to full efficiency.

ANSWERS

Line 3

An agency nurse is not in the same contractual position as the nurse employed by the health authority and the relationship between the agency and the hospital is rarely defined clearly. However, although the agency nurse in a number of ways can be categorized as self-employed, she does have an unwritten contract with the hospital to provide her services to a satisfactory standard and to abide by local policies. If an agency nurse is involved in some act that results in negligence, she may find that the health authority is unwilling to accept responsibility for her actions to the extent that it would for an employee, but it is unlikely that it can avoid vicarious liability altogether.

Line 8
The Nurses Rules 1983 state that the enrolled nurse is required to develop competencies to assist in carrying out certain functions under the direction of a registered nurse. However, an experienced enrolled nurse may be employed at a 'D' grade when she is 'expected to carry out all forms of care without direct supervision and may be required to demonstrate procedures to and supervise qualified and/or unqualified staff'. In extending the enrolled nurse's role in this way, it is to be hoped that the manager of the unit has made the necessary checks to ensure that the enrolled nurse is competent to take on this additional responsibility and that patients' safety is not put at risk.
(See Question 5.7).

Line 11
The expectations of management as to what tasks the registered nurse can undertake may well vary from one unit to another, or even between individuals. There is no clearly defined collection of skills that the nurse must acquire by law. The Nurses Rules 1983 state that certain competencies or outcomes must be achieved but these are broadly worded and will be interpreted in different ways in different settings. The profession does make certain assumptions as to what is normally accepted as inherent in the nurse's role but this may have to be clarified by looking at what is usually classed as being beyond her competency, i.e. part of an extended role.

The law becomes involved if a nurse takes responsibility for any task for which she is not adequately trained and thereby harms a patient. The law on negligence is more concerned with protecting patients than arguments as to the skill or experience of the giver of care. As was stated by Mustill L.J. in Wilsher *v*. Essex Area Health Authority 1988, the standard of care expected of the professional is that associated with the particular post and task performed rather than varying with the experience and skill of the individual.
(See Question 9.3).

Line 15
The Corruption Acts 1906 and 1916 prohibit staff from obtaining or seeking to obtain in their private or official capacity any gifts or consideration of any kind from contractors or individuals with whom they are in contact through their employment where there may be an inducement or reward for acting or refraining from acting in a certain way. Breach of these Acts could be dismissal, prosecution or, for the nurse, removal from the Register. The rule to follow is for the nurse not to accept anything which may, or may be thought likely to influence a purchasing decision. The examples given in this case study seem unlikely to be of this nature but the nurse must always be alert to the risk. The UKCC also states the professional position in the

Code of Professional Conduct Clause 13.
(See Question 6.18).

Line 20
With private care, the patient is in a contractual relationship with the hospital, unit or clinic giving the service. Therefore if there is a failure to give the service agreed, the patient can sue hospital or staff under the Supply of Goods and Services Act 1982. The National Health Service patient cannot take such action.

Line 23
Under the NHS and Community Care Act 1990, the health authority will commission services from its hospitals, NHS Trusts and general practitioners. There will then be a contractual arrangement between them for the provision of these services to certain specified and agreed standards.

Line 28
The current clinical grading structure for nurses, midwives and health visitors has clear contractual implications as to the responsibilities of the post. Within each grade, a number of criteria exist, allowing for flexibility and the reward of special skills.
(See pp. 194–196 for descriptions of clinical gradings).

Line 41
The presence of equal opportunities involves the avoidance of discrimination and there is a certain amount of legislation that is intended to prevent discrimination in relation to sex, marital status, colour and race.

The Sex Discrimination Act 1975 outlawed discrimination against either sex in applications for employment, and training and promotion prospects. However this Act does provide for a few exceptions in relation to retirement, special provisions relating to pregnancy and very occasionally specific occupations where one sex only is required for a particular job. Redress for abuse of this legislation is through the industrial tribunal system. In addition the Equal Opportunities Commission has certain powers to conduct investigations on specific employers. Often legislation on equal pay also attempts to redress inequalities between the sexes.

The Race Relations Act 1976 created the Commission for Racial Equality. The Commission has wider responsibilities than just in the area of employment but under the Act it does have powers to investigate individual employers and to draw up codes of practice for them. As with the Sex Discrimination Act, the remedy for employees is via an industrial tribunal.

Line 44
Nurses are exempt from the provisions of the Rehabilitation of Offenders Act 1974. This Act makes it lawful for people to consider their minor convictions spent after a rehabilitation period. It made it unlawful to act upon or insist upon knowledge of such convictions in relation to employ-

ment. However, certain professions which involve close contact with patients can require prospective employers to divulge such information and this is particularly important where the care of children is involved.

Line 45

It is important that prospective employers ensure that the nurse is fit to carry out the requirements of the job. The law does not lay down that a medical examination is necessary, leaving it to individual employers to decide what medical criteria to use for refusing employment. For example, a nurse with a recurrent back problem would be unlikely to be considered for work in the clinical area. The Employment Protection (Consolidation) Act 1978 does allow employment to be discontinued on the basis of incapacity due to illness (see below). However, an employer would prefer to avoid such difficulties if potential serious ill health can be predicted by pre-employment screening.
(See Question 7.4).

Line 51

An employment contract is an agreement between employer and employee and under the Employment Protection (Consolidation) Act 1978, this must be given in written form to the employee not later than 13 weeks after the commencement of employment.

Line 52

The employment contract must contain certain information again in line with the requirements of the Employment Protection (Consolidation) Act 1978. This includes the names of the parties concerned, the commencing date of employment, pay scale and intervals at which pay is received, hours of work, holiday entitlement, pension scheme, period of notice and conditions of service relating to sickness, discipline and appeals.
(See Question 9.8).

Line 58

The employee has certain minimal rights regarding pay and sickness whatever his contractual position. This involves the payment of statutory sick pay (SSP) for the first 20 weeks of sickness in any tax year, after which the responsibility for the payment of sickness benefit reverts to the Department of Social Security. However, in the National Health Service, the Whitley Council conditions give the nurse employee better benefits. For example, Roger would be due one month of full pay and one month of half pay before receiving only SSP.

Line 61

The arena of employment legislation is complex as the various statutes have to be applied in such a variety of work situations. Therefore in addition to statute law, codes of practice are developed to assist in the interpretation of the law. While these are not legally binding, they do carry a certain amount of weight in the industrial tribunal setting and certainly assist in the formulation of local policies relating to such matters as discipline, grievance and sickness. The use of these local policies is binding on the employer and employee, as they have been through a process of negotiation and agreement between management and the unions and are referred to in the contract of employment.

(See Question 5.16).

Line 62

Dismissal from employment can be fair if the employer can show what was the reason for dismissal and that this reason falls within one of those listed in the Employment Protection (Consolidation) Act 1978. One of these reasons is related to the capability of the employee to perform the work for which he has been employed and this will be assessed by reference to 'skill, aptitude, health or any other physical or mental quality'. The employer must show that he acted reasonably in treating (in this case) the sickness absence as a sufficient reason for dismissal.

(See Questions 2.17 and 9.4).

NEW CLINICAL GRADING STRUCTURE FOR NURSING AND MIDWIFERY STAFF: GRADING DEFINITIONS

Scale A

Scale A applies to posts in which the post-holder carries out assigned tasks involving direct care in support of, and supervised by, a registered nurse, midwife or health visitor.

No statutory nursing or midwifery qualifications are required for posts at this level.

Scale B

Scale B applies to posts in which the post-holder carries out assigned tasks involving direct care in support of a registered nurse, midwife or health visitor and:

a. regularly works without supervision for all or most of the shift;
b. leads a team of staff at Scale A.

No statutory nursing or midwifery qualifications are required for posts at this level.

Scale C

Scale C applies to posts in which the post-holder provides nursing care under the direction of a registered nurse, midwife or health visitor. The post-holder participates in the assessment of care needs and the implementation of programmes of care. The post-holder may be expected to demonstrate her/his own skills to new or junior members of staff.

The post-holder is normally required to have second level registration.

Scale D

Scale D applies to posts in which the post-holder is responsible for the assessment of care needs and the development of programmes of care, and/or the implementation and evaluation of these programmes. The post-holder is expected to carry out all relevant forms of care without direct supervision and may be required to demonstrate procedures to and supervise qualified and/or unqualified staff.

The post-holder is required to have:

a. first level registration;

or

b. second level registration plus a recognized post-basic certificate, or to have an equivalent level of skill acquired through experience;

or

c. second level registration and to supervise the work of other staff.

Scale E

Scale E applies to posts in which:

1. The post-holder is responsible for the assessment of care needs and the development, implementation and evaluation of programmes of care:

and

a. is expected to carry out all relevant forms of care and is designated to take charge regularly of a ward or equivalent sphere of nursing or midwifery in the absence of the person who has continuing responsibility. The post-holder is expected to supervise junior staff and be able to teach qualified and unqualified staff, including basic and/or post-basic students;

or

b. is required to have first level registration plus:

    i. a further registerable qualification;

or

    ii. a recordable post-basic certificate/statement of competence, or an equivalent level of skill acquired through experience.

or

2. The post-holder is required to take responsibility as the prime care provider for one, or a defined group of patients/mothers, in the hospital setting. He/she works with minimal supervision in the assessment of all relevant care needs, the development, implementation and evaluation of programmes of care. The post-holder is able to supervise and teach junior staff including basic and/or post-basic students.

Scale F

Scale F applies to posts in which:

1. The post-holder has continuing responsibility for the management of a ward or equivalent sphere of nursing or midwifery care, including the assessment of care needs, the development, implementation and evaluation of programmes of care, the setting of standards, and the supervision and deployment of staff; where there are no basic or post-basic students *and* where limited nursing or midwifery intervention is required.

or

2. The post-holder is responsible for the assessment of care needs, the development, implementation and

evaluation of programmes of care, without supervision, and may be required to teach other nursing and non-nursing staff.

The post-holder:

   a. is designated to take charge regularly of a ward or equivalent sphere of nursing or midwifery care in the absence of the person who has continuing responsibility and the post-holder is required to have first level registration plus:

     i. a further registerable qualification;

or

     ii. a recordable post-basic certificate/statement of competence, or equivalent level of skill acquired through experience;

or

     iii. experience in a post at Scale E;

or

   b. leads a team of staff at Grade E and below;

or

   c. undertakes duties specific to a defined client group in the community;

or

   d. is a prime care provider, who is required to practise clinical skills, developed through experience in, but more advanced than those required for, a post at Scale E.

Scale G

Scale G applies to posts in which:

1. The post-holder carries continuing responsibility for the assessment of care needs, the development, implementation and evaluation of programmes of care, and the setting of standards of care;

and

   a. the management of a ward or equivalent sphere of nursing or midwifery, including the deployment and supervision of staff, and where the teaching of students and/or extensive nursing/midwifery intervention is required;

or

   b. the management of a defined caseload, including liaison with other agencies and where appropriate the supervision, deployment and teaching of staff and/or students.

This scale is the minimum level for district nurses, community psychiatric nurses, community mental handicap nurses with the appropriate qualifications, health visitors, and midwives working in the community.

or

2. The post-holder is responsible for the management of a caseload or client group within a defined clinical area, including liaison, where appropriate, with other agencies, and the provision of specialist advice within this clinical area.

From DHSS, circular EL (88), p. 33.

RELEVANT STATUTES AND CASES

Corruption Acts 1906 and 1916
Employment Protection (Consolidation) Act 1978
NHS and Community Care Act 1990

Nurses, Midwives and Health Visitors Act 1979
Race Relations Act 1976
Rehabilitation of Offenders Act 1974
Sex Discrimination Act 1975
Supply of Goods and Services Act 1982
Cassidy *v.* Ministry of Health 1939
Wilsher *v.* Essex Area Health Authority 1988

REFERENCES

Bercusson, B. (1979) *The Employment Protection (Consolidation) Act 1978.* Sweet and Maxwell, London.

Capper, A. (1989) *Employment Legislation in Checks and Balances.* Diploma in Nursing, University of London, Unit 2 Block 5, Distance Learning Centre, South Bank Polytechnic, London.

Department of Health and Social Security (1988) *New Clinical Grading Structure for Nurses, Midwives and Health Visitors*, circular EL (88), p. 33. DHSS, London.

Rowden, R. (1987) Employment law and nurses. *Nursing* (Oxford), **3**(14), 530.

Statutory Instruments – The Nurses, Midwives and Health Visitors Rules Approval Order No. 873. 1983 HMSO, London.

Tingle, J. (1988) Negligence and Wilsher. *Solicitors Journal*, **132** (25).

UKCC (1984) *Code of Professional Conduct for Nurses, Midwives and Health Visitors.* UKCC, London.

Young, A.P. (1989) *Legal Problems in Nursing Practice*, 2nd edn. Harper and Row, London.

13 Influencing the future of health care

The topic of health and safety of both staff and patients is always of major concern and has been dealt with in earlier chapters in a number of different contexts. It is also particularly suitable when exploring how the law has changed in response to past situations and how pressure can be exerted to bring about improvements in the future.

This chapter consists of two short case studies. The issues raised are discussed at the end of each case study along with some related activities. These will assist in the application of knowledge acquired and introduce the reader to some skills needed for further study of the law.

FOOD POISONING

In August 1984 an outbreak of salmonella was confirmed at the Stanley Royd Hospital in Wakefield, a hospital for psychogeriatric patients. Both patients and staff became ill and the outbreak continued for a number of weeks. Nineteen elderly patients had died before the outbreak was over and the situation became a national scandal.

A number of factors came to light as a result of the subsequent enquiries.

The source of the outbreak was traced to infected chicken in the hospital kitchen. The old Victorian kitchen was found to be inadequate, with open drains, old equipment and poor ventilation and lighting. The situation at the Stanley Royd Hospital was not unique. The incidence of outbreaks of food poisoning and associated deaths had been a regular occurrence in hospitals, with far higher numbers than in any other public institution such as restaurants, hotels, canteens and schools. Many hospital kitchens were old with out of date equipment, ineffective cleaning, inadequate pest control, poor levels of personal hygiene amongst kitchen staff and bad practices in food preparation.

There were also criticisms at the Stanley Royd Hospital of the management of the situation at ward and nursing level. Reports at the time made allegations that ill, vomiting patients were not isolated and remained with residents who were not infected. Nurses who had themselves been sick were being allowed to return to work before

Case Studies in Law and Nursing,
Ann P. Young.
Published in 1992 by
Chapman & Hall, London
ISBN 0 412 44130 6.

stool tests had cleared them of infection and some nurses whose tests were still positive were working with instructions to avoid handling food. There was also the possibility of a lack of barrier nursing equipment and needed disinfectants being locked away.

The public enquiry laid the blame for the spread of the infection firmly at the door of local management.

COMMENTS

If the outbreak of salmonella had occurred in a school, hotel or works canteen, the management of that place could have been prosecuted and could therefore have faced severe fines. However, a hospital is Crown property and in 1984 was protected by Crown immunity from prosecution through the criminal courts. A duty of care under the law on negligence has always been applicable but requires action by a private individual rather than the State.

Therefore, the Stanley Royd Hospital management could not be prosecuted for its failure to abide by food hygiene regulations, nor for any failure to provide a safe working environment for its staff under the Health and Safety at Work (etc.) Act 1974.

The outcry about this situation put mounting pressure on the Government. In 1986, the NHS (Amendment) Act was passed. Initially the bill presented to Parliament included the lifting of Crown immunity from food hygiene laws only but a House of Lords amendment forced its extension to the Health and Safety at Work (etc.) Act 1974.

This case study is a good illustration as to how a situation can so arouse public interest and concern that a Parliamentary response follows. A brief description of how legislation comes about is given below.

Legislation

Legislation can be initiated in two ways. A Government Bill is the most usual way. Often there will be several stages prior to the publication of a bill. A Green Paper may be issued to test public opinion, followed by a White Paper which states in detail the Government's intentions in the proposed area of legislation. At both these stages, the public can comment. For example, a professional group may publish a response and communicate this to the relevant minister or member of Parliament. The other type of bill is a private member's bill. In each Parliamentary session there is a ballot as to which members of Parliament will be able to introduce a bill of their choice. Much lobbying of these MPs then takes place by various pressure groups to persuade the MP to take up their particular cause. Due to limited Parliamentary time, this latter route to legislation is only occasionally successful but may be sufficient to heighten public and political awareness of a need for legislation in a certain area, such that the matter is later incorporated in a Government Bill.

Once a bill is presented to the House of Commons in its first reading, it passes through a number of stages both within the House and in Committee where it is debated and amended. If it succeeds through these stages, it goes to the House of Lords for a similar process and once through the Lords, the bill receives the Royal Assent and becomes an Act.

Much law is now enacted via delegated legislation. This is essential in order to implement change as Parliamentary time is so limited. For example, the Health and Safety at Work (etc.) Act 1974 empowers the Health and Safety Commission to draw up regulations that are binding.

Activity 13.1

Locate a White Paper relevant to health care, for example 'Working for Patients' 1989. To what legislation did it proceed? Were there any marked changes between the White Paper and the Act?

Activity 13.2

The N.H.S. and Community Care Act 1990 Section 60 removed Crown immunity from health service bodies from 1 April 1991. This is of particular significance in relation to fire safety where a number of Acts and regulations have helped to protect the public against fire hazards but could not be enforced in the NHS prior to this date.

Building regulations control the design and construction of buildings in order to reduce the risk of fire due to the use of flammable materials and ensure the inclusion of fire-resisting measures. Buildings have to have sufficient fire exits and protected escape routes leading to a place of safety.

The Fire Precautions Act 1971 is an enabling Act which has led to the formulation of a number of Statutory Instruments with the aim of protecting life and enabling easy escape in the event of fire. Larger premises are required to obtain a fire certificate.

1. As you walk around a hospital, identify any potential fire risks and difficulties in relation to fire escapes, bearing in mind that any dangers will affect ill, not healthy, people.
2. List how much and what kind of fire training you have had. How frequently does this take place?
3. Draw up an action plan if you are concerned that fire precautions are inadequate. Chapter 7 on the Health and Safety at Work (etc.) Act 1974 may be of help here. Who can give you assistance with this task?

Activity 13.3
Find an example of a regulation implemented under the Health and Safety at Work (etc.) Act 1974 and explore the implications of this to your place of work. For example, the Control of Substances Hazardous to Health Regulations (COSHH) 1988 have important implications in the assessment of and the prevention or control of employee exposure to a range of substances.

Activity 13.4
READING A STATUTE
Part of an Act of Parliament is réproduced below. The language and layout appear confusing but if you understand its structure and follow a few simple rules in reading it, then an Act becomes much clearer. Particular points to note are numbered in the margin and explained at the end.

National Health Service (Amendment) Act 1986

1 1986, Chapter 66.

2 An Act to apply certain enactments, orders and regulations relating
3 to food and health and safety to certain health service bodies and premises; to make further provision as to pharmaceutical services under the NHS Act 1977 and the NHS (Scotland) Act 1978 and the remuneration of persons providing those services, general medical services, general dental services or general ophthalmic services under those Acts; to provide further, as respects Scotland, as to cooperation among certain bodies in securing and advancing the health of disabled persons, the elderly and others; and for connected purposes.

(7 November 1986)

4 Be it enacted by the Queen's most Excellent Majesty, by and with
5 the advice and consent of the Lords Spiritual and Temporal, and Commons, in the present Parliament assembled, and by the authority of the same, as follows:

Health and safety legislation.

6 2.-(1) For the purpose of health and safety legislation –
    (a) a health authority shall not be regarded as the servant or agent of the Crown or as enjoying any status, immunity or privilege of the Crown and
    (b) premises used by a health authority

shall not be regarded as property of
or held on behalf of the Crown.

7 ·(2) In this section
'health authority'

(a) as respects England and Wales,
has the meaning assigned to it by
Section 128 of the 1977 Act and

(b) as respects Scotland means a
Health Board constituted under
Section 2 of the 1978 Act, the
Commons Services Agency constituted
under Section 10 of that Act or a
State Hospital Management Committee
constituted under Section 91 of the
Mental Health (Scotland) Act 1984 and
'the health and safety legislation'
means

(a) the Health and Safety at Work (etc.)
Act 1974 and the regulations, orders
and other instruments in force under
it and

8 (b) the enactments specified in the
third column of Schedule 1 to that
Act and the regulations, orders and
other instruments in force under
these enactments.

·(3) Section 125 of the 1977 Act and
Section 101 of the 1978 Act shall
have no effect in relation to any
action, liability, claim or demand
arising out of the health and safety
legislation.

9 ·(4) This Section shall have no effect
in relation to anything done or
omitted before its commencement.

8.-(1) This Act may be cited as the   Short title, etc.
National Health Service (Amendment)
Act 1986.

10 (2) In this Act
'the 1977 Act' means the National Health
Service Act 1977 and
'the 1978 Act' means the National Health
Service (Scotland) Act 1978.

11 (3) Section 21(1) of the Health Services Act
1980 and paragraph 54 of Schedule 1 to that
Act shall cease to have effect.

12 (4) Sections 1 and 2 above shall come into

force at the end of the period of three
months beginning with the day on which
the Act is passed.

1. This is the short title of the Act, together with its year of publication. Sometimes the title may be further abbreviated if the
   abbreviation is well known, for example National Health Service
   to NHS.
2. This is the official citation. Each Act passed in any one year is given
   its own number and this is known as its chapter number.
3. This is the long title of the Act and gives some indication of the
   purpose behind the Act. However the long title can be misleading
   and the legal rule is that it is the main body of the Act that
   expresses the law.
4. This indicates when the Royal Assent was given and the Bill
   becomes an Act. Statutes become law on this day unless the Act
   says otherwise (see 12).
5. This is the standard form of words to show that a bill has been
   properly passed.
6. The main body of the Act is broken up into numberered sections
   and each section contains a different rule of law. By each section
   will be found marginal notes that will give a short explanation of
   the contents of that section. This helps the reader to find his
   way through an Act and clarifies the content. Each section may
   be further divided into subsections. Thus the lifting of Crown
   immunity from the health and safety legislation is found in Section
   2(1). In very long Acts, sections may be grouped together into
   parts.
7. It is important to understand the special meanings attached to
   certain words and within the Act will be sections that define and
   interpret these words.
8. Some Acts have additional schedules at the end. The contents of
   these varies. Some contain detailed provisions which are not
   found in the main body of the Act, others are reminders and
   summaries of legal rules which have been stated in the main body
   of the Act.
9. Statutes will only have a retrospective effect if this is stated in the
   Act. This section only applies after the Act becomes law.
10. See 7 above.
11. The Act spells out which sections from previous Acts are repealed
    by the Act.
12. It is important to know if an Act is not coming into force on the
    date of the Royal Assent (see 4). A commencement order has to be
    made if the Act delegates to a minister the power to decide when
    an Act will come into force. With this Act, the commencement date
    for Section 2 would have been 7 February 1987.

A BACK INJURY

The following case study is not a real case but a compilation of a number of actual incidents.

Rachel Ross was a third year student nurse when she injured her back lifting an unconscious patient up the bed. She went off sick but her injury failed to resolve with medical treatment and she had to undergo surgery 8 months after the incident. Four months later she was medically examined by the Occupational Health Department physician who advised that she was not fit to continue her nursing career. Her employment was therefore terminated.

She took advice from her union who decided to explore the possibility of negligence on the part of the health authority. There could have been negligence in a number of ways. First, the training in lifting given to Rachel could have been inadequate. Secondly, the trained nurse with whom Rachel was lifting could have failed to carry out the lift with Rachel properly, thus causing Rachel's injury. Thirdly, the employer could have failed to provide the proper resources, such as lifting equipment or adequate staff. The union's legal department decided there were grounds for proceeding and initiated an action for negligence on Rachel's behalf against the health authority.

The health authority decided to contest the action. Statements were prepared by staff who were involved in readiness for a court hearing. This eventually took place four years after the incident causing Rachel's injury.

A number of factors came to light at the hearing. There was sufficient evidence to support the health authority that training of the student had been adequate and had included information on and practice in moving an unconscious patient. There was also a hoist available on the ward. However, the lift chosen to move the patient was the Australian or shoulder lift. An expert witness, an experienced general nurse, was asked for his opinion as to the suitability of the lift in the circumstances and he stated that an unconscious patient should be lifted with at least four people and that the Australian lift was unsuitable. There was also no evidence that the trained nurse had been updated in lifting techniques since she qualified two years previously.

Rachel was awarded damages against the health authority which also had to pay costs.

COMMENTS

Both the law and accepted practice in the area of back injuries have been modified and are in the process of change as a result of a number of court cases involving injured nurses.

For many years back injuries to nurses were considered an occupational hazard about which there was little that could be done. It is only relatively recently that this attitude has changed and this has been to a large extent because certain nurses' unions have decided to take up back injuries as an important issue. It was therefore a good decision for Rachel to involve her union.

Another important point in gaining the support of a union is that of cost. The price of legal advice is considerable and once barristers become involved, the costs escalate rapidly. There is a system of legal aid for those on very low incomes, but most individuals in employment would not be able to apply for this. A sizeable proportion of those with a potentially good case are deterred from suing as they could lose thousands of pounds in costs if they did not win. The financial and legal support of a union has ensured that a number of cases involving back injured nurses have been heard, with the result that judges have been able to interpret the law on negligence in this area.

In Rachel's case, the union decided to sue the health authority rather than individual members of staff. This gave Rachel's lawyers the freedom to explore a number of possible areas of negligence as explained in the case study and is possible as the health authority has to accept vicarious liability for the wrongs of its employees.

Once a case comes to court, it can influence the law in a number of ways. In this case study, an expert witness gave evidence as to the accepted manner of moving an unconscious patient. This expert opinion of what constitutes accepted professional practice has played an important part in medical and nursing cases. In R. *v.* Arthur 1981 (summarized in Chapter 10), expert witnesses supported as established practice Dr Arthur's decision to sedate and give water only to a newborn baby with Down's syndrome. This certainly influenced the final acquittal of Dr Arthur of attempted murder.

All law has to be interpreted in a variety of situations and certain court cases can influence later cases by means of precedents. A precedent is a previous decision of a court which may in certain circumstances be binding on another court in deciding a similar case (the law in Scotland also uses certain legal principles). It depends on the level of the court as to which decisions are binding on future cases. In most situations the case has to be heard at an appeal court or higher. One case affecting back injured nurses was Williams *v.* Gwent HA 1982 which set a precedent that even if an employee uses a wrong lifting technique it is up to the employer to ensure that the employee uses the correct method.

The amount of damages may also be influenced by previous cases. Initially awards were low but as the number of cases coming before the courts increased so have the awards. At the time of going to print, the record award is £184,603 (McGowan *v.* Harrow HA 1991).

Activity 13.5

Some discussion took place in Chapter 2 as to how to write a statement. The points to remember are repeated below in more detail. Study them and then write a statement of some incident that you have been involved in that may have later repercussions, for example a drug error, a patient complaint or an accident. In reality, you would be wise to ask for assistance or for a more experienced person to look at what you have written before submitting the statement.

1. Include full name, status and length of time employed in the post.
2. Identify the relevant period of duty, when it started and if there was anything exceptional about it.
3. Introduce those involved in the incident including physical or mental state if this is relevant.
4. Describe the sequence of events. Try to state accurate times if possible.
5. Explain why you took the actions you did. This may include saying why you did not take certain actions.
6. Report conversations in direct speech to avoid ambiguity.
7. Use clear language and avoid words you do not understand. Avoid abbreviations and check that spelling is correct.
8. If an error has been made and you acknowledge this, then include any mitigating circumstances, for example staff shortage, emergencies. Do not try to cover up for other people's mistakes.
9. Every word you write must be true. Avoid assumptions, hearsay and emotive statements.
10. Only include relevant material and be reasonably concise without losing the sense of what happened.
11. Number each page and sign it at the bottom. Date and sign the statement immediately below the text.
12. Reread the statement after a break. Any corrections should also be signed. Keep a copy.

Activity 13.6

In order to find out about recent changes in the law, carry out a media watch for several weeks. Nursing journals carry brief comments of some cases and statutory changes and longer reports are found in the *Times*, *Independent* and *Guardian* newspapers. If you have access to a legal section of a college library, cases are reported in the weekly Law Reports and the All England Law Reports.

Note the status of the court hearing a case as this has an effect on whether the case will create a legal precedent or not. Figures 13.1 and 13.2 demonstrate the hierarchy of the courts.

(a) Civil Courts

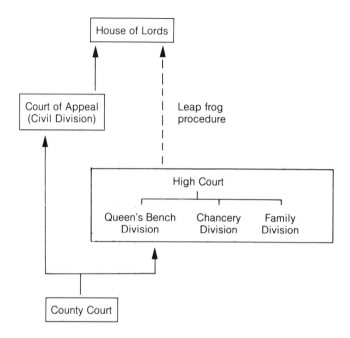

(b) Criminal Courts

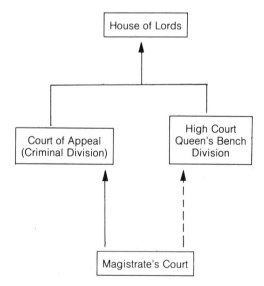

Fig. 13.1 The courts in England, Wales and N. Ireland.

(a) Civil Courts

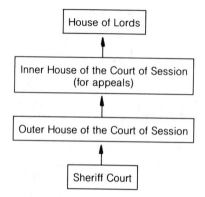

(b) Criminal Courts

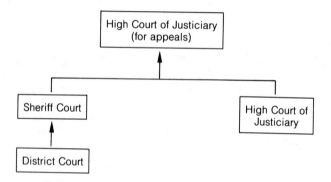

Fig. 13.2 The courts in Scotland.

Activity 13.7

The increase in cases involving back injured nurses has not only influenced case law. Health authorities have responded by improving safety in this area, the motivation probably being to reduce litigation costs! Responses from the Health and Safety Commission and Executive have also occurred.

Explore what policies and practices exist in your health authority in relation to lifting and handling patients. Have guidelines and regulations been produced under the Health and Safety at Work (etc.) Act 1974?

RELEVANT STATUTES

Fire Precautions Act 1971
Health and Safety at Work (etc.) Act 1974
National Health Service (Amendment) Act 1986
National Health Service and Community Care Act 1990

REFERENCES

Beckett, A. and Young, A. (1989) Health and safety at work, in *Checks and Balances*, Diploma in Nursing, University of London, Unit 2 Block 5, Distance Learning Centre, South Bank Polytechnic, London.

Bradney, A. *et al.* (1986) *How to Study Law*. Sweet and Maxwell, London.

Brown, P. (1990) How to state your case. *Nursing Times*, **86**(38), 52–4.

Health and Safety Commission (1989) *Control of Substances Hazardous to Health Regulations*. HMSO, London.

Nursing Times (1984) Food poisoned nurses back to work too soon, say unions. 12 September, p. 5.

Pritchard, J. (1984) *Guide to the Law*. Penguin, Harmondsworth, Middlesex.

Rogers, R. and Salvage, J. (1988) *Nurses at Risk*. Heinemann, London.

Salvage, J. (1985) *The Politics of Nursing*. Heinemann, London.

White Paper (1989) *Working for Patients*. HMSO, London.

Young, A.P. (1989) *Legal Problems in Nursing Practice*, 2nd edn. Harper and Row, London.

Young, A.P. (1991) *Law and Professional Conduct in Nursing*. Scutari, London.

Appendix A

Nurses, midwives and health visitors (training amendment rules) approval order 1989 no. 1456

PREPARATION FOR ENTRY TO PARTS 12, 13, 14 AND 15 OF THE REGISTER

18A-(2) The Common Foundation Programme and the Branch Programme, shall be designed to prepare the student to assume the responsibilities and accountability that registration confers, and to prepare the nursing student to apply knowledge and skills to meet the nursing needs of individuals and of groups in health and in sickness in the area of practice of the Branch Programme and shall include enabling the student to achieve the following outcomes:

  (a) the identification of the social and health implications of pregnancy and child bearing, physical and mental handicap, disease, disability, or ageing for the individual, her or his friends, family and community;

  (b) the recognition of common factors which contribute to, and those which adversely affect, physical, mental and social well-being of patients and clients and take appropriate action;

  (c) the use of relevant literature and research to inform the practice of nursing;

  (d) the appreciation of the influence of social, political and cultural factors in relation to health care;

  (e) an understanding of the requirements of legislation relevant to the practice of nursing;

  (f) the use of appropriate communication skills to enable the development of helpful caring relationships with patients and clients and their families and friends, and to initiate and conduct therapeutic relationships with patients and clients;

  (g) the identification of health-related learning needs of patients and clients, families and friends and to participate in health promotion;

  (h) an understanding of the ethics of health care and of the nursing profession and the responsibilities which these

Case Studies in Law and Nursing,
Ann P. Young.
Published in 1992 by
Chapman & Hall, London
ISBN 0 412 44130 6.

impose on the nurse's professional practice;

(i) the identification of the needs of patients and clients to enable them to progress from varying degrees of dependence to maximum independence, or to a peaceful death;

(j) the identification of physical, psychological, social and spiritual needs of the patient or client; an awareness of values and concepts of individual care; the ability to devise a plan of care, contribute to its implementation and evaluation; and the demonstration of the application of the principles of a problem solving approach to the practice of nursing;

(k) the ability to function effectively in a team and participate in a multi-professional approach to the care of patients and clients;

(l) the use of the appropriate channel of referral for matters not within her sphere of competence;

(m) the assignment of appropriate duties to others and the supervision, teaching and monitoring of assigned duties.

Appendix B

Summary of questions and activities by chapter

1 RESPECTING THE INDIVIDUAL

Questions

1.1 Right of entry to person's home.
1.2 Abiding by patient's wishes *re* contacting GP – confidentiality.
1.3 Breach of confidentiality – doctor talking to relatives, patient preventing this.
1.4 Grounds for admission against patient's wishes – arranged by family.
1.5 Patient advocacy – patient's wishes contrary to family.
1.6 Property on admission.
1.7 Data Protection Act 1984.
1.8 Prevention of patient leaving hospital – not under Section but confused.
1.9 Use of restraint with confused patient.
1.10 Duty of witness to accidents *re* the police.
1.11 Making a statement to the police.
1.12 Giving treatment without consent – a confused patient.
1.13 Necessity of involving patient in planning care – ownership of documents and consent.
1.14 Decision on when patient is to be discharged.
1.15 Home help and district nurse legislation.
1.16 Property on discharge.
1.17 Do professionals know best?

Activities

1.1 Legal entitlement to enter a patient's home.
1.2 UKCC leaflet, *Confidentiality*, pp. 3–7.
1.3 Local policy and documentation on property.
1.4 Maintaining confidentiality of nursing and medical records.
1.5 List of ways a patient may be restrained.
1.6 Analysis of a statement made to the police.
1.7 Format of care plans and patient access to them.
1.8 Arranging district nurse and home help services on discharge.

2 SAFETY OF PATIENTS AND COLLEAGUES

Questions

2.1 Importance of documenting a patient's assessment – possible negligence, etc.
2.2 Consent of spouse when patient unconscious.
2.3 Accusations of maltreatment (link with assessment).
2.4 Accidents to patients – reason for accident form – negligence.
2.5 Follow-up observations after an accident – refuting negligence.
2.6 Reasons for staff accident form.
2.7 Faults in completing an accident form.
2.8 Health and Safety at Work (etc.) Act 1974 – back injuries.
2.9 Drug error and negligence – preventing harm.
2.10 Importance of drug and disciplinary policies *re* safe care.
2.11 Legal requirement *re* frequency of documenting care.
2.12 How to document care in a legally useful way.
2.13 Patient smoking and safety – possible negligence.
2.14 Requiring visitors to leave the ward – trespass.
2.15 Risk taking and negligence *re* accidents.
2.16 Chronically Sick and Disabled Persons Act 1970 – aids and modifications in the home.
2.17 Dismissal from job because of sickness.

Activities

2.1 Wording on Accident and Emergency and ward assessment forms.
2.2 Patient accident forms in use.
2.3 Where drug and disciplinary policies are kept and read drug policy.
2.4 Care plans available to you.
2.5 Health authority rules *re* visitors, particularly children.
2.6 Occupational health regulations *re* nurses and infection risks.

3 COMMUNICATING WITH PATIENTS, RELATIVES AND COLLEAGUES

Questions

3.1 Police and the MHA – place of safety.
3.2 Refusal to treat in the A and E Dept – potential negligence.
3.3 Asking for help – acknowledging limitations (negligence).
3.4 Preventing a patient leaving A and E Dept – MHA, negligence.
3.5 Emergency admission – MHA.
3.6 Information sharing – patient going from A and E Dept to ward.
3.7 Justification of sedating a patient without consent (MHA).

3.8   Getting information about a patient from another hospital – ownership of notes.

3.9   How to delegate care without negligence.

3.10 Patient choice *re* personal cleanliness – safety of others.

3.11 Assessment of student nurses – negligence to patients, employment factors.

3.12 Legal justification for lying – consent.

3.13 Responsibilities of psychiatrist, social worker and nurse towards mentally ill.

3.14 Consent and the informal patient.

3.15 Nurses' role in advising doctor *re* treatment.

3.16 Information given to relatives over the telephone.

3.17 Discharge against a patient's/relative's wishes.

3.18 Dealing with complaints.

Activities

3.1   Formal admissions, MHA.

3.2   Patient rights under the MHA.

3.3   Rights laid down in practical assessment procedures.

3.4   UKCC leaflet, *Exercising Accountability*, pp. 10–11.

3.5   UKCC leaflet, *Administration of Medicines*, Section 4a–i.

3.6   Local complaints procedure.

4 WORKING IN THE COMMUNITY

Questions

4.1   Community nurse accepting patient's key – trespass, theft.

4.2   Disabled access to buildings.

4.3   Disabled and housing.

4.4   Occupiers' liability in the home *re* equipment.

4.5   Refusal to give care in order to protect self from harm (occupiers' liability).

4.6   Back injury in patient's home.

4.7   Disabled and employment.

4.8   Grounds for abortion.

4.9   Maternity leave.

4.10 Child minding.

4.11 Duty to assist at accident in the street – professional discipline.

4.12 Duty of care of nurse at accident in street – negligence.

4.13 Documenting failure to give care – avoiding negligence.

4.14 Avoiding negligence when inexperienced.

4.15 Workloads in the community – negligence.

4.16 Precautions to avoid violence in the street.

4.17 Responsibilities of health authority *re* community staff and violence – health and safety at work.

4.18 Refusal to visit patients in the community – personal safety.
4.19 Legislation and suspected child abuse.
4.20 Visiting a patient's home if violence threatened – occupiers' liability.

Activities

4.1 Access for disabled in shopping centre.
4.2 Maintenance of equipment in the patient's home.
4.3 Numbers of disabled employed in health authority and in what jobs.
4.4 Creche facilities.
4.5 Police advice to community nurses.
4.6 Comparison of community and hospital nursing documents.

5 WORKING IN AN INSTITUTION

Questions

5.1 Definitions of mental handicap.
5.2 Mentally handicapped – whose responsibility?
5.3 Assuming consent (mentally handicapped).
5.4 Negligence and a wet bed.
5.5 Questioning decision making between two poor alternatives – assault or negligence.
5.6 Duty to update knowledge and skills – negligence.
5.7 Obedience to seniors – justification for refusal.
5.8 Supervision of student by unqualified staff, potential negligence of qualified staff.
5.9 Legal requirements of checking drugs.
5.10 Reporting misconduct of a colleague.
5.11 Shopping and lending patients money.
5.12 Suspected theft by a patient from other patients.
5.13 Failing to give information to staff – potential negligence.
5.14 Definition of libel.
5.15 Grounds against a successful action for libel.
5.16 Value of joining a union or professional body.
5.17 Responsibility for students in the clinical area.
5.18 Griffiths community report.

Activities

5.1 Patterns/models of nursing in use in the health authority.
5.2 UKCC leaflet, *Administration of Medicines*, Section 4g and h.
5.3 Financial arrangements for longstay patients in hospital.
5.4 Unions and professional bodies available for nurses and what benefits they offer.
5.5 Criteria for accepting a clinical area for nurse training.
5.6 Making a grievance, local grievance policy.

6 STANDARDS OF CARE

Questions

6.1   Blood tests and consent.
6.2   Overhearing of confidential information.
6.3   Informing a patient of diagnosis – nurse's role.
6.4   Misconduct and breach of contract – disciplinary measures.
6.5   Safety on a paediatric ward – negligence.
6.6   Child's right to information.
6.7   Nurse's role *re* giving a patient information.
6.8   Age of consent of child.
6.9   Overruling parents' refusal to give consent.
6.10 Medical research and experiments – consent, negligence.
6.11 Participation of relatives in patient's care – negligent delegation.
6.12 Injuries to visitors – occupiers' liability.
6.13 Legal precautions and nursing research – negligence, discipline.
6.14 Implementing change through formal channels – policy formation.
6.15 Extended role of the community nurse – legal requirements.
6.16 Negligence or unavoidable risks of treatment.
6.17 Giving wrong advice/information and negligence.
6.18 Receiving gifts.

Activities

6.1   UKCC leaflet, *Confidentiality*, pp. 8–9.
6.2   UKCC professional conduct committee – reasons for appearance.
6.3   Safety in an area where children are kept.
6.4   Patient safety and drug trials.
6.5   UKCC Code of Professional Conduct.

7 ADULT NURSING

Questions

7.1   Legal controls of AIDS and HIV.
7.2   Refusal to give care – reasons, outcomes.
7.3   Health and safety at work – infections.
7.4   Employment and HIV infections.
7.5   Patient's refusal to give consent.
7.6   Hastening a patient's death.
7.7   Nurse's role *re* gaining consent and giving information.
7.8   Following patient's wishes once unable to give consent.
7.9   Failure to initiate resuscitation.
7.10 Legal definition of death.
7.11 Property at death.
7.12 Death and the coroner.

Activities

7.1 Control of infection policy.
7.2 Staff policy *re* HIV screening.
7.3 UKCC leaflet, *Exercising Accountability*.
7.4 Visit a coroner's court.

8 MENTAL HEALTH NURSING

Questions

8.1 Legal detention in hospital.
8.2 Section 2 admission.
8.3 Patient's rights under Section.
8.4 Attempted suicide and negligence.
8.5 Information *re* medication (patient under Section).
8.6 Rehabilitation and negligence.
8.7 Relatives and the MHA.
8.8 Patient's refusal to see a visitor.
8.9 Nurse's holding power under the MHA.
8.10 Nurse injured by violent patient.
8.11 Drug compliance after discharge.

Activities

8.1 Role of the CPN.
8.2 Forms 2 and 3, MHA.
8.3 Safety features in the psychiatric ward.
8.4 Section 5 MHA forms.

9 MENTAL HANDICAP NURSING

Questions

9.1 LA responsibility *re* housing for mentally handicapped.
9.2 Refusal of consent by mentally handicapped.
9.3 Nurses Rules Section 18A.
9.4 Nurse violence against a patient, possible outcomes.
9.5 Relative making a complaint.
9.6 Employment, education and training for the mentally handicapped.
9.7 Protection and freedom for the mentally handicapped.
9.8 Job changes and contractual implications.
9.9 Nurses' professional and friendship roles.

Activities

9.1 UKCC disciplinary procedures.
9.2 Visit industrial tribunal or UKCC professional conduct committee hearing.
9.3 Facilities for mentally handicapped in colleges.

10 CHILDREN'S NURSING

Questions

10.1 Notification and registration of births.
10.2 The law and the seriously handicapped baby.
10.3 Scarce resources in the Health Service.
10.4 Organ donation.
10.5 Parents' legal rights and responsibilities.
10.6 Removal of parental responsibilities.
10.7 Legal aspects of information issues.
10.8 Discontinuing life support systems.
10.9 Negligence in the operating theatre.
10.10 Lay people's access to medical information.

Activities

10.1 Waiting lists in the health authority.
10.2 The donor card.
10.3 Prevention of accidents in the operating theatre.

Appendix C

Summary of questions by main topic areas

ABORTION

4.8 Grounds for abortion.
7.2 Conscientious objection.

ADMISSION

1.4 Admission against patient's wishes.
3.5 Emergency admission, MHA.
Activity 3.1 Formal admission, MHA.
8.2 MHA Section 2 Admission.
8.3 Patient's rights under section.

BIRTHS

10.1 Notification and registration of births.
10.2 The seriously handicapped baby.

COMMUNITY LEGISLATION

1.15 Home help and district nurse legislation.
Activity 1.8 Arranging home help and district nurse services on discharge.
2.16 Chronically Sick and Disabled Persons Act 1970 – aids and modifications in the home.
4.2 Disabled access to buildings.
4.3 Disabled and housing.
4.7 Disabled and employment.
4.10 Child minding.
4.19 Legislation and suspected child abuse.
5.2 Responsibility for mentally handicapped.
5.18 Griffiths community report.
9.1 LA responsibilities *re* housing for mentally handicapped.
9.6 Employment, education and training for mentally handicapped.
10.6 Removal of parental responsibilities.

COMPLAINTS

3.18 Dealing with complaints.
9.5 Relative making a complaint.

CONFIDENTIALITY

1.2   Abiding by patient's wishes *re* GP.
1.3   Breach of confidentiality – doctor and relatives.
1.7   Data Protection Act.
Activity 1.2 UKCC *Confidentiality* leaflet, pp. 3–7.
6.2   Overhearing of confidential information.
Activity 6.1 UKCC *Confidentiality* leaflet, pp. 8–9.
10.7 Legal aspects of information issues.

CONSENT

1.5   Patient advocacy – patient's wishes contrary to family.
1.12 Giving treatment without consent – a confused patient.
1.13 Involving patient in planning care.
2.2   Consent when patient unconscious.
3.7   Sedating patient without consent (MHA).
3.10 Patient choice and personal cleanliness.
3.12 Legal justification for lying.
3.14 Consent and the informal patient.
5.3   Assuming consent (mentally handicapped).
6.1   Blood tests.
6.8   Age of consent of child.
6.9   Overruling parents' refusal to give consent.
6.10 Consent – medical research, experiments.
7.5   Patient's refusal to give consent.
7.8   Following patient's wishes once unable to give consent.
8.11 Drug compliance after discharge.
9.2   Refusal of consent by mentally handicapped.
10.5 Child's degree of choice.

DEATH AND DYING

7.6   Hastening a patient's death.
7.9   Failure to initiate resuscitation.
7.10 Legal definition of death.
7.12 Death and the coroner.
10.2 The law and the seriously handicapped baby.
10.4 Organ donation.
10.8 Discontinuing life support systems.

DETENTION IN HOSPITAL

1.8   Confused patient.
3.4   A and E Dept.
8.1   Legal detention in hospital.

DISCHARGE

1.13 Failure to gain patient's cooperation leading to self-discharge.
1.14 Decision on when patient to be discharged.
3.17 Discharge against a patient's/relative's wishes.

DISCIPLINE AND PROFESSIONAL CONDUCT

2.10 Importance of disciplinary policies for safe care.
5.7   Obedience to seniors, justification for refusal.
5.10 Reporting misconduct of a colleague.
6.4   Misconduct and breach of contract – disciplinary measures.
Activity 6.2 Reasons for appearance at UKCC professional conduct com-
              mittee.
7.2   Refusal to give care – reasons, outcomes.
9.4   Nurse violence against a patient.
Activity 9.1   UKCC disciplinary procedures.

DOCUMENTATION

1.13 Planning patient care – ownership of documents.
Activity 1.7 Format of care plans, patient access to them.
2.1   Importance of documenting patient's assessment.
2.4   Reason for accident form (patients).
2.6   Reasons for staff accident form.
2.7   Faults in completing an accident form.
2.11 Frequency of documenting care.
2.12 How to document care in a legally useful way.
Activity 2.1 Wording of assessment forms.
          2.2 Patient accident forms.
          2.4 Care plans.
4.13 Documenting failure to give care.
Activity 4.6 Community and hospital nursing documents.

DRUGS

2.9   Drug error.
2.10 Importance of drug policy.
Activity 2.3 Read drug policy.
5.9   Legal requirements of checking drugs.
Activity 5.2 UKCC *Administration of Medicines* leaflet, Section 4g and h.

Activity 6.4 Drug trials.
7.6   Hastening a patient's death.
8.11 Drug compliance after discharge.

EMPLOYMENT LEGISLATION

2.17 Dismissal from job because of sickness.
4.9   Maternity leave.
5.16 Value of joining a union or professional body.
Activity 5.4 Benefits of unions and professional bodies available to nurses.
6.14 Policy formation.
9.4   Dismissal because of misconduct.
9.8   Job changes and contractual implications.
9.9   Nurses' professional roles.
12   Whole chapter.

HEALTH AND SAFETY AT WORK

2.8   Back injuries.
Activity 2.6 Occupational health regulations *re* nurses and infection risks.
4.6   Back injury in patient's home.
4.16 Avoiding violence in the streets.
4.17 Responsibilities of HA *re* community staff and violence.
4.18 Personal safety and refusal to visit patients in the community.
Activity 4.5   Police advice to community nurses.
7.1   Legal control of AIDS and HIV.
7.3   Infections and health and safety.
7.4   Employment and HIV infections.
8.10 Nurse injured by violent patient.

INFORMATION GIVING/SHARING

1.2   Contacting the GP.
1.3   Doctor talking to relatives.
3.3   Asking for help, acknowledging limitations.
3.6   Information sharing – patient from A and E Dept to ward.
3.8   Getting information about a patient from another hospital, ownership of notes.
3.12 Lying.
3.13 Responsibilities of different staff towards mentally ill.
3.15 Nurses' role in advising doctor.
3.16 Information given over the telephone.
Activity 3.2 Leaflet *Your rights under the Mental Health Act 1983*.
5.13 Failing to give information to staff.
5.14 Definition of libel.
5.15 Grounds against a successful action for libel.
6.3   Nurse's role in informing patient of diagnosis.

6.6   Child's right to information.
6.7   Nurse's role in giving patient information.
6.17   Giving wrong advice/information.
7.7   Nurse's role *re* gaining consent.
8.5   Giving information *re* medication.
10.7   Legal aspects of information issues.
10.10 Lay people's access to medical information.

MENTAL HEALTH ACT

1.4   Grounds for admission against patient's wishes.
3.1   Police and place of safety.
3.5   Emergency admission.
3.7   Sedating patient without consent.
3.13   Responsibilities of psychiatrist, social worker and nurse.
Activity 3.1 Formal admissions.
Activity 3.2 Patients' rights.
5.1   Definitions of mental handicap.
7.5   Patient's refusal to give consent.
8.1   Legal detention in hospital.
8.2   Section 2 admissions.
8.3   Patient's rights under Section.
8.7   Relatives and the MHA.
8.9   Nurse's holding power under the MHA.
8.11   Drug compliance after discharge.
Activity 8.2 Forms 2 and 3, MHA.
Activity 8.4 Section 5 forms.

NEGLIGENCE

1.8   Prevention of confused patient leaving hospital.
2.1   Documenting a patient's assessment.
2.3   Accusations of maltreatment.
2.4   Accidents to patients.
2.5   Follow-up observations after an accident.
2.9   Drug error and negligence.
2.13   Patient smoking and safety.
2.15   Risk taking and negligence.
3.2   Refusal to treat in the A and E Dept.
3.4   Preventing a patient leaving the A and E Dept.
3.9   Delegating care without negligence.
3.11   Assessment of student nurses, negligence to patients.
4.12   Duty of care of nurse at accident.
4.13   Documenting failure to give care.
4.14   Avoiding negligence when inexperienced.
4.15   Workloads in the community.
5.4   Negligence and a wet bed.

5.5   Decision making between two poor alternatives.
5.6   Duty to update knowledge and skills.
5.8   Supervision of students.
5.13   Failing to give information to staff.
6.5   Safety on a paediatric ward.
6.10   Medical research and experiments.
6.11   Delegation of patient's care to relatives.
6.13   Nursing research.
6.15   Extended role of the community nurse.
6.16   Negligence or unavoidable risks of treatment.
6.17   Giving wrong advice/information.
7.2   Refusal to give care.
8.4   Attempted suicide and negligence.
8.6   Rehabilitation and negligence.
9.7   Protection and freedom for the mentally handicapped.
10.3   Scarce resources in the National Health Service.
10.9   Negligence in the operating theatre.

OCCUPIER'S LIABILITY

4.4   Equipment in the home.
4.5   Refusal to give care in order to protect self from harm.
4.20   Violence threatened in a patient's home.
6.12   Injuries to visitors.

POLICE

1.1   Right of entry to person's home.
1.10   Duty of witness to an accident.
1.11   Making a statement to the police.
Activity 1.6 Analysis of a statement.
3.1   Police and the MHA.
Activity 4.5 Police advice to community nurses.
5.12   Suspected theft by a patient.

PROPERTY

1.6   On admission.
1.16   On discharge.
5.11   Shopping and lending patients money.
5.12   Suspected theft.
Activity 5.3 Financial arrangements for longstay patients.
6.18   Receiving gifts.
7.11 At death.

RESTRAINT

1.9   Use of restraint with confused patient.
Activity 1.5 Ways a patient may be restrained.
8.9   Nurse's holding power under the MHA.
8.10 Violent patient.

TRESPASSERS, VISITORS

1.1   Right of entry into person's home.
2.14 Requiring visitors to leave the ward.
4.1   Community nurse accepting patient's key.
4.20 Visiting a patient's home.
8.8   Patient's refusal to see a visitor.

VIOLENCE

4.16 Avoiding violence in the street.
4.17 Responsibilities of health authority *re* community staff and violence.
4.20 Violence threatened in patient's home.
8.10 Nurse injured by violent patient.
9.4   Nurse violence against a patient.

Appendix D

UKCC booklets

CODE OF PROFESSIONAL CONDUCT
FOR THE NURSE, MIDWIFE AND HEALTH VISITOR

Each registered nurse, midwife and health visitor shall act, at all times, in such a manner as to justify public trust and confidence, to uphold and enhance the good standing and reputation of the profession, to serve the interests of society, and above all to safeguard the interests of individual patients and clients.

Each registered nurse, midwife and health visitor is accountable for his or her practice, and, in the exercise of professional accountability shall:

1. Act always in such a way as to promote and safeguard the well being and interests of patients/clients.
2. Ensure that no action or omission on his/her part or within his/her sphere of influence is detrimental to the condition or safety of patients/clients.
3. Take every reasonable opportunity to maintain and improve professional knowledge and competence.
4. Acknowledge any limitations of competence and refuse in such cases to accept delegated functions without first having received instruction in regard to those functions and having been assessed as competent.
5. Work in a collaborative and co-operative manner with other health care professionals and recognise and respect their particular contributions within the health care team.
6. Take account of the customs, values and spiritual beliefs of patients/clients.
7. Make known to an appropriate person or authority any conscientious objection which may be relevant to professional practice.
8. Avoid any abuse of the privileged relationship which exists with patients/clients and of the privileged access allowed to their property, residence or workplace.
9. Respect confidential information obtained in the course of professional practice and refrain from disclosing such information without the consent of the patient/client, or a person entitled to act on his/her behalf, except where disclosure is required by law or by the order of a court or is necessary in the public interest.

10. Have regard to the environment of care and its physical, psychological and social effects on patients/clients, and also to the adequacy of resources, and make known to appropriate persons or authorities any circumstances which could place patients/clients in jeopardy or which militate against safe standards of practice.

11. Have regard to the workload of and the pressures on professional colleagues and subordinates and take appropriate action if these are seen to be such as to constitute abuse of the individual practitioner and/or to jeopardise safe standards of practice.

12. In the context of the individual's own knowledge, experience, and sphere of authority, assist peers and subordinates to develop professional competence in accordance with their needs.

13. Refuse to accept any gift, favour or hospitality which might be interpreted as seeking to exert undue influence to obtain preferential consideration.

14. Avoid the use of professional qualifications in the promotion of commercial products in order not to compromise the independence of professional judgement on which patients/clients rely.

Notice to all registered nurses, midwives and health visitors

This Code of Professional Conduct is issued by the United Kingdom Central Council for Nursing, Midwifery and Health Visiting.

It is issued for the guidance and advice of all registered nurses, midwives and health visitors.

Further explanatory notes, discussion papers or comments on specific points in the Code of Professional Conduct may be issued by the Council from time to time.

The Code will be subject to periodic review by the Council.

The Council expects members of the profession to recognise it as their responsibility (as well as the Council's) to re-appraise the relevance of the Code to the professional and social context in which they practice.

The Council will welcome suggestions and comments for consideration in its periodic review of the Code of Professional Conduct. Such suggestions and comments should be sent to:

United Kingdom
Central Council
for Nursing,
Midwifery and
Health Visiting
(PC Division)
23 Portland Place
London W1N 3AF

CONFIDENTIALITY
A UKCC ADVISORY PAPER

An elaboration of Clause 9 of the Second Edition of the UKCC's Code of Professional Conduct for the Nurse, Midwife and Health Visitor.
    A framework to assist individual professional judgement.
    The contents of this Advisory Paper apply to all persons whose names appear on any part of the Professional Register maintained by the UKCC and to those undertaking courses of education and training with a view to admission to the Register.
    It is essential that the document be read from its beginning to understand properly the issues addressed.

A. Introduction

1. The Code of Professional Conduct for the Nurse, Midwife and Health Visitor (Second Edition) published by the United Kingdom Central Council for Nursing, Midwifery and Health Visiting is

   a statement to the profession of the primacy of the interests of the patient or client;

   one of the principal means by which the Council is seeking to comply with Section 2(5) of the Nurses, Midwives and Health Visitors Act 1979 and give advice to its practitioners on standards of professional conduct;

   a portrait of the practitioner the Council believes to be needed and wishes to see within the profession.

2. In approving the terms of this edition of the Code the Council authorised the publication of key statements on a number of important professional issues.

3. One of these key statements (Clause 9) concerns 'Confidentiality'. It reads: –

   'Each registered nurse, midwife and health visitor is accountable for his or her practice, and, in the exercise of professional accountability shall:
   Respect confidential information obtained in the course of professional practice and refrain from disclosing such information without the consent of the patient/client, or a person entitled to act on his/her behalf, except where disclosure is required by law or by the order of a court or is necessary in the public interest.'

4. It can be seen from the general description of the Code of Professional Conduct and the particular contents of Clause 9 that breaches of confidentiality should be regarded as exceptional, only occurring after careful consideration and the exercise of personal professional judgement.

5. Any codified statements of this nature need continuous exploration, and on occasions a more detailed and authoritative elaboration. It is for the

whole profession to recognise its responsibility to share in such exploration, to use the respective knowledge and skill of practitioners to facilitate it and to recognise the important contribution the professional press makes to this essential debate. The subject of confidentiality has emerged as one on which the profession's practitioners need the relevant clause in the Code of Professional Conduct to be developed more fully by the UKCC. It must be said, however, that no exploration or elaboration by others alters the fact that the ultimate decision is that of the individual practitioner in the situation. The demand for elaboration of Clause 9 of the Code has focused particularly on determining the difficult boundary that applies in any case between the expectations of patients/clients that information, whether recorded or not, obtained in the course of profession practice will not be disclosed, and the expectations of the public that they will not be put at risk because practitioners unreasonably withhold information.

It is not the purpose of this document to seek to provide answers to the many dilemmas which practitioners face. It is necessary, however, to provide examples of them since they have been a backcloth against which the discussions culminating in the publication of this document have taken place.

Correspondence on this point has come (for example) from: –

a sister in a psychiatric day hospital who found a patient possessed of large quantities of controlled drugs that he cannot have obtained legally;

a medical practitioner concerned that a community midwife reported to her employers the fact that while visiting the wife of a hospital employee in a professional capacity she saw substantial quantities of stolen hospital property;

a health visitor who has been told by one child that another child is being sexually abused;

Accident and Emergency Department nursing staff who found that the unconscious patient they were treating had a gun on his person;

nurses working in the community who have been instructed by their managers (following approval by an ethical committee) to give researchers direct access to confidential information in respect of patients, but who knew that the consent of those patients had not been sought;

psychiatric nurses who fear that information revealed by a patient in a therapeutic group may be passed on by other patients and that the nurses will be held responsible;

occupational health nurses faced with requests from their managers for information about employees;

community psychiatric nurses who were reluctant to comply with the instruction to put full names and addresses of patients visited on their travel expense claims;

a health visitor who had become aware that information she shared with a social worker in a case conference had been given in evidence in a Magistrates' Court;

practitioners who have chosen not to make a record of information given to them by patients in confidence, and who have later been worried about the propriety of their decision; and

a health authority chairman who asks 'Who is to define the public interest?' and 'How is the nurse to recognise the authenticity of the claim of public interest?'

The Council has been left in no doubt that it has a responsibility to address this important subject in greater depth.

As already stated, the UKCC is not seeking to provide responses to those dilemmas since a judgement must be made by the individual practitioner concerned. It is instead seeking to provide guidance on disclosure of information:

(a) to assist development of understanding about the nature and scope of the dilemma which practitioners face, and to encourage those who employ nurses, midwives and health visitors to recognise the difficult and stressful situations encountered by practitioners and to offer support and guidance, stimulate discussion and develop and publicise policies on this important matter;

(b) to state certain principles which it is hoped will assist practitioners to consider situations which they encounter and to make sound professional judgements;

(c) to emphasise that the responsibility of whether or not information should be withheld or disclosed without the consent of the patient/client lies with the practitioner involved at the appropriate time and cannot be delegated;

(d) to stress that those who employ or supervise nurses, midwives and health visitors have an obligation to support these practitioners in discharging their responsibilities in respect of the right to disclose or withhold information using their professional judgement;

(e) to indicate the conditions which should be met before disclosure of information, so that the decision to either disclose or withhold information can be justified.

B. Defining terms

1. What do we mean when we speak of something being 'Confidential'? Turn to almost any Dictionary and you find that the focal word in the definitions of 'confide', 'confidence' or 'confidential' is 'TRUST'. To trust another person with private and personal information about yourself is a significant matter. Where the person to whom that information is given is a nurse, midwife or health visitor the patient/client has a right to believe that this information, given in confidence in the expectation that it will be used only for the purposes for which it was given, will not be released to

others without the consent of the patient/client. The death of a patient/ client does not absolve the practitioner from this obligation.

2. Clearly it is impractical to obtain the consent of the patient/client every time that health care information needs to be shared with other health professionals, or other staff involved in the health care of that patient/ client. Consent in these instances can be implied provided that it is known and understood by the patients/clients that such information needs to be made available to others involved in the delivery of his/her care. Patients/clients have a right to know the standards of confidentiality maintained by those providing their care, and these standards should be made known by the health professional at the first point of contact. These standards of confidentiality can be reinforced by the additional use of leaflets and posters where the health care is being delivered.

3. When an individual practitioner considers that it is necessary to obtain the explicit consent of a patient/client before disclosing specific information, it is the responsibility of the practitioner to ensure that the patient/client can make as informed a response as possible as to whether that information can be disclosed or withheld.

4. It is essential that nurses, midwives and health visitors recognise the fundamental right of their patients or clients to information about them being kept private and secure. This point is sharply reinforced by only brief consideration of the personal, social or legal repercussions which might follow unauthorised disclosure of information concerning a person's health or illness.

5. Disclosure of information occurs in the following ways:
   (a) with the consent of the patient/client;
   (b) without the consent of the patient/client when the disclosure is required by law or order of a court;
   (c) by accident;
   (d) without the consent of the patient/client when the disclosure is considered necessary in the public interest.

   It is the latter two categories that this Advisory Paper is particularly addressing, for a breach of confidentiality occurs if anyone deliberately or by accident gives information, which has been obtained in the course of professional practice, to a third party without the consent of the patient/ client.

6. The public interest, in the context of this Advisory Paper, is taken to mean the interests of an individual, of groups of individuals or society as a whole, and would (for example) encompass matter such as serious crime, child abuse and drug trafficking.

C. Ownership and care of confidential information

1. The organisations which employ professional practitioner staff who make records (whether in the National Health Service or in other spheres of practice) are the legal owner of such records, but such ownership does not give them any legal right of access to the information contained in

those records. The patient also is involved in the ownership. The ownership of a record is therefore irrelevant to the patient's right of confidentiality and his/her expectation that identifiable personal health information will not be disclosed without consent.

2. In many situations genuine difficulties can be experienced in preventing the leakage of confidential information or its inadvertent spread into management layers leading to possible misuse. There is need for particular caution where a system of shared records is employed, it being incumbent on the author of any particular entry to satisfy himself or herself that other people with access to that shared record will respect the confidentiality of the information and will place neither the patient/client nor the author of the entry at risk by its release without consent.

3. The task with which individual professional practitioners are faced is not limited to that of exercising a judgement as to what information can be or should be disclosed. It also includes that of ensuring or helping to ensure that record keeping systems are not such as to make the release of information possible or likely. Neither technology nor management convenience should be allowed to determine principles. Each practitioner has a responsibility to recognise that risks exist, and to satisfy himself or herself in respect of the system for storage and movement of records operated in the health care setting in which he or she works and to ensure that it is secure. The concern for the environment of care for which each practitioner is held accountable under the terms of clause 10 of the Code of Professional Conduct for the Nurse, Midwife and Health Visitor extends to include this.

4. The practitioner should act so as to ensure that he/she does not become a channel through which confidential information obtained in the course of professional practice is inadvertently released. The dangerous consequences of careless talk in public places cannot be overstated.

5. Where access to the records of patients or clients is necessary so that students may be assisted to achieve the necessary knowledge and competence it must be recognised that the same principles of confidentiality stated earlier in this document extend to them and their teachers. The same applies to those engaged in research. It is incumbent on the practitioner(s) responsible for the security of the information contained in these records to ensure that access to it is closely supervised, and occurs within the context of the teacher and student undertaking to respect its confidentiality, and in knowledge of the fact that the teacher has accepted responsibility to ensure that students understand the requirement for confidentiality and the need to observe local policies for the handling and storage of records. It is expected that the student or teacher who is active in giving care as a practitioner will apprise the patient of their role, thus enabling the patient who is so capable to control the information flow. Where deemed necessary the recipient of confidential information from a patient/client will advise him/her that the information will be conveyed to the nurse, midwife or health visitor involved in his/her care on a continuing basis.

6. It is advisable that the contracts of employment of all employees not directly involved with patients/clients but who have access to or handle confidential records contain clauses which emphasise the principles of confidentiality and state the disciplinary consequences of breaching them. Paragraph 3.20 of the Report from the Confidentiality Working Group of the DHSS Steering Group on Health Services Information suggests a form of words worthy of consideration as follows:

> 'In the course of your duties you may have access to confidential material about patients, members of staff or other health service business. On no account must information relating to identifiable patients be divulged to anyone other than authorised persons, for example medical, nursing or other professional staff, as appropriate, who are concerned directly with the care, diagnosis and/or treatment of the patient. If you are in any doubt whatsoever as to the authority of a person or body asking for information of this nature you must seek advice from your superior officer. Similarly, no information of a personal or confidential nature concerning individual members of staff should be divulged to anyone without the proper authority having first been given. Failure to observe these rules will be regarded by your employers as serious misconduct which could result in serious disciplinary action being taken against you, including dismissal.'

The circumstances in which a nurse, midwife or health visitor chooses to disclose or withhold confidential information are explored in Section D.

D. Deliberate breach of confidentiality in the public interest or that of the individual patient/client

1. The examples given in paragraph A5 remind us that we live in a real world, and that sometimes there are a range of interests to consider.

   Pressure is often exerted on practitioners to breach the principle of keeping confidential and maintaining the security of information elicited from patients/clients in the privileged circumstances of a professional relationship. This should not be regarded as surprising, since 'Confidentiality' is a rule with certain exceptions. There is no statutory right of confidentiality; but there is also no bar to an aggrieved individual bringing a common law case before a civil court alleging breach of confidentiality and seeking financial recompense.

   It is essential that before determining that a particular set of circumstances constitute such an exception, the practitioner must be satisfied that the best interests of the patient/client are served thereby or the wider public interest necessitates disclosure.

2. The needs of the community can, on occasions, take precedence over the individual's rights as for example in those situations where a Court rules that the administration of justice demands that a professional confidence be broken or the law requires that patient confidence be breached.

3. In many other situations sharing of confidential information occurs by intention. This is the case where information obtained in the course of professional practice is shared with other professionals in the health and social work fields in the belief that to do so is in the interests of the patient/client. Legislation concerned with data protection and its associated codes is not intended to prevent the exchange of information between professional staff who share the care of the patient/client. It is, however, the duty of the practitioner who obtains and holds the information to ensure, as far as is reasonable, before its release that it is being imparted in strict professional confidence and for a specific purpose. The same duty applies where the practitioner is contributing to a shared record. Wherever possible the consent of the patient/client to the sharing of information should first be obtained.

4. The situations that are the most exceptional and problematic for the practitioner are those where the deliberate decision to withhold confidential information or disclose it to a third party can have very serious consequences. The information can have been given to the practitioner in the strictest confidence or the practitioner may have obtained the information inadvertently in the course of his or her professional practice. The decision as to whether to make a record of such information, like the decisions as to whether or not to disclose, poses many dilemmas, for the situations are invariably complex. In some instances the practitioner can be under pressure to divulge information but it must be emphasised that the responsibility lies with him or her as an individual. This responsibility cannot be delegated.

5. In all cases where the practitioner deliberately discloses or withholds information in what he/she believes the public interest he/she must be able to justify the decision. These situations can be particularly stressful, especially where vulnerable groups are concerned, as disclosure may mean the involvement of a third party as in the case of children or the mentally handicapped. Practitioners should always take the opportunity to discuss the matter fully with other practitioners (not only or necessarily fellow nurses, midwives and health visitors), and if appropriate consult with a professional organisation before making a decision. There will often be ramifications and these are best explored before a final decision as to whether to withhold or disclose information is made.

Once having made a decision the practitioner should write down the reasons either in the appropriate record or in a special note that can be kept on file. The practitioner can then justify the action taken should that subsequently become necessary, and can also at a later date review the decision in the light of future developments.

E. Summary of the principles on which to base professional judgement in matters of confidentiality

1. That a patient/client has a right to expect that information given in confidence will be used only for the purpose for which it was given and will not be released to others without their consent.

2. That practitioners recognise the fundamental right of their patients/ clients to have information about them held in secure and private storage.

3. That, where it is deemed appropriate to share information obtained in the course of professional practice with other health or social work practitioners, the practitioner who obtained the information must ensure, as far as is reasonable, before its release that it is being imparted in strict professional confidence and for a specific purpose.

4. That the responsibility to either disclose or withhold confidential information in the public interest lies with the individual practitioner, that he/she cannot delegate the decision, and that he/she cannot be required by a superior to disclose or withhold information against his/her will.

5. That a practitioner who chooses to breach the basic principle of confidentiality in the belief that it is necessary in the public interest must have considered the matter sufficiently to justify that decision.

6. That deliberate breaches of confidentiality other than with the consent of the patient/client should be exceptional.

The UKCC members and officers responsible for the preparation of this document greatly appreciate the opportunity afforded them to discuss it in its formative stages with representatives of the General Medical Council.

ADMINISTRATION OF MEDICINES
A UKCC ADVISORY PAPER

A framework to assist individual professional judgement and the development of local policies and guidelines.

Introduction

1. The framework which is set out in this document should be considered against the background of the extracts from Statutory Instrument 1983 No. 873 (The Nurses, Midwives and Health Visitor Rules) and the UKCC Code of Professional Conduct for the Nurse, Midwife and Health Visitor which are reproduced for convenience, and of the definitions given for the terms 'professional judgement' and, 'professional responsibility'.

2. It is intended for practitioners of nursing, midwifery and health visiting wherever they are practising. The main body of the text relates to 'normal' circumstances. Guidelines in respect to exceptional circumstances are set out in an Appendix to the main document.

3. The relevant primary legislation concerning the administration of medicines is the Medicines Act, 1968, and the Misuse of Drugs Act, 1971.

4. The term 'medicine' refers to controlled drugs and 'prescription only' medicines as defined in those Acts. It includes 'General Sales List' medicines in those settings where they are normally subject to prescription.

5. Wherever in this paper the word 'practitioner' is used it refers to a practitioner of nursing, midwifery or health visiting.
6. This advisory document is released following helpful consultation with the General Medical Council and the Pharmaceutical Society.

Background

1. Rule 18 of Statutory Instrument 1983 No. 873 states: –
Courses leading to a qualification the successful completion of which shall enable an application to be made for admission to Part 1, 3, 5 or 8 of the register shall provide opportunities to enable the student to accept responsibility for her personal professional development and to acquire the competencies required to: –
(a) advise on the promotion of health and the prevention of illness;
(b) recognise situations that may be detrimental to the health and well-being of the individual;
(c) carry out those activities involved when conducting the comprehensive assessment of a person's nursing requirements;
(d) recognise the significance of the observations made and use these to develop an initial nursing assessment;
(e) devise a plan of nursing care based on the assessment with the co-operation of the patient, to the extent that this is possible, taking into account the medical prescription;
(f) implement the planned programme of nursing care and where appropriate teach and co-ordinate other members of the caring team who may be responsible for implementing specific aspects of the nursing care;
(g) review the effectiveness of the nursing care provided, and where appropriate, initiate any action that may be required;
(h) work in a team with other nurses, and with medical and para-medical staff and social workers;
(i) undertake the management of the care of a group of patients over a period of time and organise the appropriate support services;
related to the care of the particular type of patient with whom she is likely to come in contact when registered in that Part of the register for which the student intends to qualify.
Courses leading to a qualification the successful completion of which shall enable an application to be made for admission to Part 2, 4, 6, or 7 of the register shall be designed to prepare the student to undertake nursing care under the direction of a person registered in Part 1, 3, 5 or 8 of the register and provide opportunities for the student to develop the competencies required to: –
(a) assist in carrying out comprehensive observation of the patient and help in assessing her care requirements;
(b) develop skills to enable her to assist in the implementation of

nursing care under the direction of a person registered in Part 1, 3, 5 or 8 of the register;

(c) accept delegated nursing tasks;

(d) assist in reviewing the effectiveness of the care provided;

(e) work in a team with other nurses, and with medical and paramedical staff and social workers;

related to the care of the particular type of patient with whom she is likely to come into contact when registered in that Part of the register for which the student intends to qualify.'

2. The different but quite specifically stated competencies in Rule 18(1) for the nurses whose names appear in the first level parts of the register (i.e. Registered General Nurse, Registered Mental Nurse, Registered Nurse of the Mentally Handicapped, Registered Sick Children's Nurse), and in Rule 18(2) for the nurses whose names appear in the second level parts of the register (i.e. Enrolled Nurse, General; Enrolled Nurse, Mental; Enrolled Nurse, Mental Handicap; Enrolled Nurse) should be noted.

3. In relation to the administration of medicines, the midwife has the same responsibility as the first level nurse.

4. The UKCC Code of Professional Conduct for the Nurse, Midwife and Health Visitor contains the following important statements: –

Each registered nurse, midwife and health visitor shall act, at all times, in such a manner as to justify public trust and confidence, to uphold and enhance the good standing and reputation of the profession, to serve the interests of society, and above all to safeguard the interests of individual patients and clients.

Each registered nurse, midwife and health visitor is accountable for his or her practice, and, in the exercise of professional accountability shall:

(i) act always in such a way as to promote and safeguard the well being and interests of patients/clients;

(ii) ensure that no action or omission on his/her part or within his/her sphere of influence is detrimental to the condition of safety or patients/clients;

(iii) take every reasonable opportunity to maintain and improve professional knowledge and competence;

(iv) acknowledge any limitations of competence and refuse in such cases to accept delegated functions without first having received instruction in regard to those functions and having been assessed as competent;

5. For the purpose of this advisory paper the following definitions are drawn to your attention: –

(i) Professional Judgement in health care is personal judgement based on special knowledge and skill, and always and above all is exercised in the best interests of the patient/client.

(ii) Professional Responsibility in health care is personal responsibility based on special knowledge and skill for actions, attitudes and policies always and above all directed to the best interests of the patient/client.

The framework

1. TREATMENT WITH MEDICINES

The treatment of a patient with medicines for therapeutic, diagnostic or preventative purposes is a process which involves prescribing, dispensing, administering and receiving.

The word 'patient' is used since any person receiving a prescribed medicine is the patient of that prescriber at the time of prescription.

2. PRESCRIBING (THE DOCTOR'S ROLE)

(a) This involves obtaining a patient's consent (commonly this is implicit) based on an understanding of the treatment, and issuing a prescription written legibly, indelibly and dated. The prescription must ensure accurate patient identification, specify the preparation to be given and where appropriate its form (e.g. tablets, capsules, suppositories, etc) and strength, the dose, the timing and frequency of administration and the route of administration. In the case of patients for whom a prescription is provided in the Out-Patient or Community setting, the number of dose units or total course must be stated.

(b) In the case of controlled drugs, the dose must be written in words and figures and in the Out-Patient or Community setting the total dose or number of dose units in both words and figures to be supplied, the whole being in the prescriber's own handwriting.

(c) Prescriptions must be signed and dated by the prescribing doctor.

(d) There are certain situations (e.g. in Registered Nursing Homes) where a medicine will have to be administered against a prescription which is no longer available. Unless the prescription was very specific the container will probably bear the instruction to administer 'as directed' only. In such circumstances the prescribing doctor should produce a written order against which medicines can be checked.

(e) Any practitioner faced with a prescription not satisfying the above criteria should withhold administration and request the doctor concerned to write a full and correct prescription. (See paragraph 4(c) on page 240).

(f) The administration of medicines on verbal instruction except in emergencies does not satisfy acceptable criteria.

(g) Instruction by telephone to a nurse to administer, even in an emergency situation, a hitherto unprescribed drug cannot be supported. This practice is unreliable and involves a nurse in a procedure which is potentially hazardous to the patient. This paragraph must, however, be read in the context of the supplementary advice set out in the appendix to this document on pages 242 and 243.

(h) Where it is the wish of the doctors that nursing staff be authorized to administer certain medicines such as mild analgesics, laxatives and topical applications a local protocol which satisfies the general criteria of the appendix to this paper should be agreed between the medical, nursing and pharmaceutical professionals involved.

(i) The exemptions for midwives and occupational health nurses under the terms of the Medicines Act 1968 and the Misuse of Drugs Act 1971 and subsequent regulations are referred to in paragraph 4(1) on page 241.

3. DISPENSING (THE PHARMACIST'S ROLE)

(a) This involves checking that the prescription is written correctly to avoid misunderstanding or error, appropriate in the circumstances, and that any newly prescribed medicine will not dangerously interact with or nullify the effect of any previously prescribed medicines or food.

(b) In addition the pharmacist is involved in determining quality, advising on security and storage conditions, compounding the medicine in a form suitable for administration to the relevant patient, providing relevant additional information on container labels and annotating the prescription to render it accurate.

(c) Still further the pharmacist is involved in monitoring the adverse side effects of medicines, and should therefore be sent any information which the administering practitioner deems relevant.

(d) It should be noted that amendments to a prescription which are made and signed by the pharmacist after consultation with the prescribing doctor are acceptable.

(e) When the pharmacist is satisfied on all appropriate points, his/her role further involves clear labelling, insertion into an appropriate container and secure delivery.

4. ADMINISTERING (THE ROLE OF THE NURSE, MIDWIFE AND HEALTH VISITOR)

(a) The exercise of professional judgement (which involves the application of his/her knowledge and experience to the situation faced) will lead the practitioner to satisfy himself/herself that he/she is competent to administer the medicine and prepared to be accountable for that action. Once that decision has been made, the practitioner follows a sequence of steps to ensure the safety and well being of the patient, and which must as a prerequisite be based on a sound knowledge of the patient's assessment and the environment in which care is given.

(b) Correctness

This involves interpretation of the prescription and container information in terms of what has been prescribed. Illegibility and lack of clarity of the instruction must be questioned. It also involves ensuring that the medicine is to be administered to the patient for whom it has been prescribed, and in the form and by the method prescribed.

Certain of these points do not usually apply in the context of a patient's home where the patient is receiving medicines from a personalised container. The visiting practitioner does, however, have a responsibility to assist the patient's understanding and help ensure safe administration.

Where a patient is in possession of a range of medicines in containers which are not labelled with precise instructions, and the danger of over or under administration exists, it may be necessary for the practitioner to advise the prescribing doctor so that he/she may consider whether any action is required.

(c) Appropriateness and the possible need to withhold

This involves checking the expiry date of the medicine, careful consideration of the dosage and the method, route and timing of administration in the context of the condition of each specific patient. It may be necessary or deemed advisable at the time when a medicine is due to be administered to withhold it in order to seek further verification from the prescribing doctor, or confirmation from the responsible senior nurse that it should be given. Where, in the opinion of the administering nurse or responsible senior nurse, (i.e. the nurse on duty to whom the administering nurse is in line responsibility at the time) contra-indications to the administration of the medicine are observed the prescribing doctor should be contacted without delay.

(In respect of this point and that at (b) above the advice of the relevant pharmacist will often be helpful in those situations where the prescribing doctor or an appropriate alternative doctor cannot be contacted.)

(d) Reinforcement

The positive effect of treatment may need to be reinforced by the nurse. Every occasion on which a medicine is administered is an opportunity for such reinforcement and for reassurance. In the community particularly it is also an opportunity to help ensure avoidance of misuse of self-medication, and the misuse of the prescribed drugs by others who reside in or are visiting the household.

(e) Recording/Reporting

As part of the ongoing process (not solely at the times of administration of medicines) the effects and side-effects of the treatment should be noted. Taking appropriate action in relation to side-effects is essential. Positive and negative effects should be reported to the appropriate doctor and recorded.

(f) Record of Administration

Where a practitioner is involved in the administration of medicines thorough and accurate records of the administration must be maintained. In hospital settings this will normally be achieved by initialling the appropriate box on a treatment record at the time of administration. Otherwise the date and time of administration, together with the administering practitioner's signature are essential minimum requirements, and all must be legibly written. If (as a result of consideration as in 'c' above) a medicine is not administered a record to that effect should be made.

(g) The UKCC is of the view that practitioners whose names are on the first level parts of the register, and midwives, should be seen as competent to administer medicines on their own, and responsible for their actions in so doing. The involvement of a second person in the administration of medicines with a first level practitioner need only occur where that practitioner is instructing a learner or the patient's condition makes it necessary or in such other circumstances as are locally determined.

Where two persons are involved responsibility still attaches to the senior person.

(h) The UKCC is totally opposed to the involvement of personnel who are not professionally registered such as nursing auxiliaries or assistants in the administration of medicines since it gives a false sense of security, undermines true responsibility, and fails to satisfy points (c) and (d) of this section.

(i) Given the wording of Rule 18(2) of Statutory Instrument 1983 No. 873, the UKCC is opposed to the use of a second level practitioner for the administration of medicines other than under the direction of a first level nurse. It is recommended that employers adopt the same stance unless: –

   (1) they have provided additional instruction relevant to the medicines likely to be encountered in a particular setting;

   (2) they have undertaken an assessment of the individual's knowledge and competence to perform the task; and

   (3) they are prepared to accept the responsibility for any errors that are consequential upon using a second level practitioner beyond the role for which training prepared him/her. (See BACKGROUND 1 and 2 of this paper).

(j) The principles enunciated in this section are equally applicable to a medicine round or to the administration of medicines within individual care.

(k) The responsibility of the nurse varies in the setting of a patient's home, where he/she needs to be cognizant of the 'freedom' of the patient in his own setting, and the implications of self-medication and the possession of 'over the counter' medicines. Where a nurse working in the community becomes involved in obtaining prescribed medicines for patients he/she must recognise his/her responsibility for their safe transit and correct delivery.

(l) In accordance with the requirements of the Medicines Act 1968 and the Misuse of Drugs Act 1971 and subsequent regulations there are specific arrangements for midwives working in the community, and occupational health nurses, to obtain and administer medicines. Those relating to midwives are contained in the UKCC Midwife's Code of Practice and those to occupational health nurses in the Royal College of Nursing Society of Occupational Health Nursing Information Leaflet No. 11 dated November 1983. Also in pursuance of Regulation 10(3) of the Misuse of Drugs Regulations 1973 specific 'Group Authority' is given to certain registered nurses employed at places of work.

5. RECEIVING (THE PATIENT'S ROLE)

The patient's role is as participant. The point of receiving provides the opportunity for: –

(a) Validation

   Ensuring that the patient understands the treatment, the need to complete the prescribed course and has consented to receiving it.

(b) Education/Instruction

Assessing and promoting the patient's knowledge and understanding regarding his/her medication, and reinforcing safety; this is essential before the patient can progress to independence. The role of the relatives and other informal carers is an important consideration in the rehabilitation of the patient.

(c) Self-Administration

Monitoring the patient's self-administration of prescribed medicines (where the practice is established) or preparing the patient for self-administration at home or in hospital as part of a planned programme towards independence. At home and at work account must be taken of the possibility of self-medication with non-prescribed medicines.

6. THE LEGISLATIVE ASPECT

Medicinal products are subject to legislative controls relating to their manufacture, prescription, sale, handling, storage and custody. The nurse therefore operates within a legal framework in respect of: –

(a) Supplies. Proper procedures should be employed for ordering. Checking deliveries and maintaining records are key factors. Orders should not be such that stocks will be excessive and wastage likely.

(b) Storage. As well as being kept in a secure place as required by legislation, drugs should be stored in the appropriate environment as instructed by the respective manufacturers.

(c) Stocktaking. This involves recording, checking stocks and disposing of unwanted medicines according to legislation. Discrepancies in stocks must be reported and investigated.

Collaborative working with the Pharmacist will ensure that appropriate systems are developed in respect of these three important aspects of the process aimed at safe administration of medicines.

Supplement suggesting variations which should apply where the specific framework is not appropriate

(a) There are certain situations in which practitioners are involved in the administration of medicines where specific factors within the preceding framework are difficult to apply or could not be applied without introducing dangerous delay and its consequent risk to patients.

(b) These will include occupational nursing settings in industry, small hospitals with no resident medical staff and possibly some specialist units within larger hospitals and a variety of community settings.

(c) In any situations in which practitioners may be expected or required to administer 'prescription only' medicines to patients which have not been directly prescribed for those patients by a medical practitioner who has examined and made a diagnosis, it is essential that a clear policy be determined which enables action to be taken in the patients' interests and to protect the practitioners from risk of complaint which might jeopardise their employment or professional status.

(d) It is therefore recommended that, in any situation where practitioners might be called upon or expected to administer 'prescription only' medicines which have not been directly prescribed as a result of examination, the following principles should be agreed and set down in a local policy which is known to all practitioners likely to be involved.

(i) It should first be agreed and then set down in writing by all the doctors working within a particular setting that there are circumstances in which particular 'prescription only' medicines may be administered in advance of examination by a doctor. Where frequent staff changes make this impractical one senior doctor should be appointed by his/her colleagues to establish such policies on their behalf, with them undertaking to honour his/her decision. A review of such policies must take place annually.

(ii) The particular circumstances in which a particular 'prescription only' medicine (and its form, route, etc.) could be administered must then be the subject of specific and well documented agreement, which must have similar support.

Wherever possible agreements should, in the particular organisation to which they apply, satisfy the needs likely to emerge in paragraph 2(g) on page 238.

(iii) Except where there is an appropriate senior nurse to provide this instruction it must be the responsibility of one of the doctors working in the setting (acting on behalf of all the doctors) or, where appropriate, a pharmacist to undertake instruction of any practitioner who will be expected to administer any 'prescription only' medicine which has not been specifically prescribed, this instruction to encompass information concerning the medicine, the indications for its use, its effects and side-effects, and any contra-indications. Where an appropriate senior nurse is available for this purpose he/she must not hesitate to call upon the services of the doctor, especially in relation to aspects of diagnosis, pharmacology and prescribing.

(iv) The above instruction should conclude with an assessment of knowledge and competence which is a necessary prelude to the preparation of the written document authorising a particular practitioner to administer a particular 'prescription only' medicine without a specific prescription in a particular set of circumstances.

(v) No practitioner should be expected to accept the responsibility for administering such medicines against his/her will, and those who do accept the responsibility must remember the requirements of the UKCC Code of Professional Conduct that they acknowledge any limitations in their competence and seek appropriate instruction.

(e) Practitioners who engage in the administration of 'prescription only' medicines which have not been specifically prescribed for a particular patient following medical examination and diagnosis in any situation where the above 5 criteria have not been fully met are rendering themselves extremely vulnerable. However, where these criteria are

fully satisfied the nurse would normally be protected from the consequences of his or her actions even if made the subject of a complaint to
the Statutory Regulating Bodies.

EXERCISING ACCOUNTABILITY
A UKCC ADVISORY DOCUMENT

A framework to assist nurses, midwives and health visitors to consider
ethical aspects of professional practice.

This is the 4th document in a series to supplement the Code of Professional Conduct for the Nurse, Midwife and Health Visitor. (Second Edition;
November 1984).

In the text that follows the use of the feminine gender equally implies the
male and similarly the use of the male gender equally implies the female.

The word 'Practitioner' in this document means a registered nurse,
midwife or health visitor. Where reference is made to a practitioner from
another profession it is indicated by the relevant prefix.

The contents of this Advisory Paper are relevant to all persons whose
names appear on any part of the Professional Register maintained by the
UKCC and will be of special interest to those undertaking courses of
education and training with a view to admission to the Register.

In order to understand fully the issues addressed it is essential that the
advisory paper should be read in its entirety.

A. *Introduction*

1. The United Kingdom Central Council for Nursing, Midwifery and Health
   Visiting regulates the nursing, midwifery and health visiting professions
   in the public interest.

   The UKCC was established by the Nurses, Midwives and Health Visitors
   Act 1979.

   Section 2(1) of the Nurses, Midwives and Health Visitors Act 1979 states
   that 'The principal functions of the Central Council shall be to establish
   and improve standards of training and professional conduct'.

   Section 2(5) of the same Act moves from the requirement to improve
   conduct to one of the methods to be employed when it states that 'The
   powers of the Council shall include that of providing in such manner as
   it thinks fit, advice for nurses, midwives and health visitors on standards
   of professional conduct'.

2. The Code of Professional Conduct for the Nurse, Midwife and Health
   Visitor is the Council's definitive advice on professional conduct to its
   practitioners. In this extremely important document practitioners on the
   UKCC's register find clear and unequivocal statements as to what their
   regulatory body expects of them. It therefore also provides the backcloth
   against which any alleged misconduct on their part will be judged.

   The Code of Professional Conduct is considered to be

a statement to the professional of the primacy of the interests of the patient or client.

a statement of the profession's values.

a portrait of the practitioner which the Council believes to be needed and which the Council wishes to see within the profession.

3. The Council has already published three advisory documents to supplement the Code of Professional Conduct. Practitioners now seek:
   (i) elaboration of clauses 10 & 11 of the Code and support for their position when doing as these clauses require. These Clauses state that: –

   'Each registered nurse, midwife and health visitor is accountable for his or her practice and, in the exercise of professional accountability, shall: –

   10. Have regard to the environment of care and its physical, psychological and social effects on patients/clients, and also to the adequacy of resources, and make known to appropriate persons or authorities any circumstances which could place patients/clients in jeopardy or which militate against safe standards of practice.
   11. Have regard to the workload of and the pressures on professional colleagues and subordinates and take appropriate action if these are seen to be such as to constitute abuse of the individual practitioner and/or to jeopardise safe standards of practice'.

   (ii) advice and guidance on issues related to consent and the general subject of truth telling.
   (iii) advice and guidance on that part of the practitioner's role which concerns advocacy on behalf of patients and clients.
   (iv) elaboration of clause 5 of the Code which states that each registered nurse, midwife and health visitor shall:

   5. 'Work in a collaborative and co-operative manner with other health care professionals and recognise and respect their particular contributions within the health care team'.

   (v) advice and guidance on issues related to contentious treatments and conscientious objection.

   This document provides a response to those requests, aims to assist professional practitioners to exercise their judgement and reinforces the importance of the Code of Professional Conduct.

B. The Code of Professional Conduct and the subject of accountability

1. This new UKCC advisory document has been produced in order to establish more clearly the extent of accountability of registered nurses,

midwives and health visitors and to assist them in the exercise of professional accountability in order to achieve high standards of professional practice.

2. The Code begins with an unequivocal statement

> 'Each registered nurse, midwife and health visitor shall act, at all times, in such a manner as to justify public trust and confidence, to uphold and enhance the good standing and reputation of the profession, to serve the interests of society, and above all to safeguard the interests of individual patients and clients'.

This introductory clause indicates that a registered practitioner is accountable for her actions as a professional at all times, whether engaged in current practice or not and whether on or off duty.

In situations where the practitioner is employed she will be accountable to the employer for providing a service which she is employed to provide and for the proper use of the resources made available by the employer for this purpose.

In the circumstances described in the preceding two paragraphs the practitioner has an ultimate accountability to the UKCC for any failure to satisfy the requirements of the introductory paragraph of the Code of Professional Conduct.

The words 'accountable' and 'accountability' each occur only once in the Code, both being found in the stem paragraph out of which the subsequent 14 clauses grow. They do, however, provide its central focus as the Code is built upon the expectation that practitioners will conduct themselves in the manner it describes.

3. Accountability is an integral part of professional practice, since, in the course of that practice, the practitioner has to make judgements in a wide variety of circumstances and be answerable for those judgements. The Code of Professional Conduct does not seek to state all the circumstances in which accountability has to be exercised, but to state important principles.

The primacy of the interests of the public and patient or client provide the first theme of the Code and establish the point that, in determining his or her approach to professional practice, the individual nurse, midwife or health visitor should recognise that the interests of public and patient must predominate over those of practitioner and profession. The second major theme is the exercise by each practitioner of personal professional accountability in such a manner as to respect the primacy of those interests.

4. The Code of Professional Conduct states unequivocally that all practitioners who are registered on the UKCC's register are required to seek to set and achieve high standards and thereby to honour the requirement of Clause 1 of the Code which states that each registered nurse, midwife and health visitor shall: –

1. 'Act always in such a way as to promote and safeguard the wellbeing and interests of patients and clients'.

It is recognised that, in many situations in which practitioners practice, there may be a tension between the maintenance of standards and the availability or use of resources. It is essential, however, that the profession, both through its regulatory body (the UKCC) and its individual practitioners, adheres to its desire to enhance standards and to achieve high standards rather than to simply accept minimum standards. Practitioners must seek remedies in those situations where factors in the environment obstruct the achievement of high standards: to start from a compromise position and silently to tolerate poor standards is to act in a manner contrary to the interests of patients or clients, and thus renege on personal professional accountability.

C. *Concern in respect of the environment of care*

1. The dilemma for practitioners in many settings in respect of the environment of care is very real and has been well documented. If practitioners express concern at the situations which obstruct the achievement of satisfactory standards they risk censure from their employers. On the other hand, failure to make concerns known renders practitioners vulnerable to complaint to their regulatory body (the UKCC) for failing to satisfy its standards and places their registration status in jeopardy.

   The sections of the Code of Professional Conduct that are particularly relevant to this issue are the introductory paragraphs and clauses numbered 1, 2, 3, 10 & 11. These parts of the Code apply to each and every person on the Council's register. Whether engaged in direct care of the patient or client, or further removed but in a position to exert influence over the setting in which that contact exists, the practitioner is subject to the Code and has an accountability for her actions or omissions.

2. The import of the Sections of the Code referred to is that, having, as part of her professional accountability, the responsibility to 'serve the interests of society and above all to safeguard the interests of individual patients and clients' and to 'act always in such a way as to promote and safeguard the wellbeing and interests of patients/clients', the registered nurse, midwife and health visitor must make appropriate representations about the environment of care: –
   (a) where patients or clients seem likely to be placed in jeopardy and/or standards of practice endangered;
   (b) where the staff in such settings are at risk because of the pressure of work and/or inadequacy of resources (which again places patients at risk); and
   (c) where valuable resources are being used inappropriately.
   This is an essential part of the communication process that should operate in any facility providing health care, to ensure that those who determine, manage and allocate resources do so with full knowledge of the consequences for the achievement of satisfactory standards. Nurses, midwives and health visitors in management positions should ensure that all relevant information on standards of practice is obtained and com-

municated with others involved in health policy and management in the interests of standards and safety.

3. Practitioners engaged in direct patient or client care should not be deterred from making representations of their concerns regarding the environment of care simply because they believe that resources are unavailable or that action will not result. The immediate professional manager to whom such information is given, having assessed that information, should ensure that it is communicated to more senior professional managers. This is important in order that, should complaints be made about the practitioners involved in delivering care, the immediate and senior managers will be able to confirm that the perceived inadequacies in the environment of care have been drawn to their attention.

It is clearly wrong for any practitioner to pretend to be coping with the workload, to delude herself into the conviction that things are better than they really are, to aid and abet the abuse and breakdown of a colleague, or to tolerate in silence any matters in her work setting that place patients at risk, jeopardise standards of practice, or deny patients privacy and dignity.

In summary, Section C of this document simply restates the UKCC's expectations (set out in the Code of Professional Conduct) that while accepting their responsibilities and doing their best to fulfil them, practitioners on its register will ensure that the reality of their clinical environment and practice is made known to and understood by appropriate persons or authorities, doing this as an expression of their personal professional accountability exercised in the public interest. An essential part of this process is the making of contemporaneous and accurate records of the consequences for patients and clients if they have not been given the care they required.

4. The Code of Professional Conduct applies to all persons on the Council's register irrespective of the post held. Their respective will vary with their role, but they share the overall responsibility for care. No practitioner will find support in the Code or from the UKCC for the contention that genuinely held concerns should not be expressed or, if expressed, should attract censure.

D. Consent and truth

1. It is self-evident that for it to have any meaning consent has to be informed. For the purposes of this document "informed consent" means that the practitioner involved explains the intended test or procedure to the patient without bias and in as much detail (including detail of possible reactions, complications, side effects and social or personal ramifications) as the patient requires. In the cases of an unquestioning patient the practitioner assesses and determines what information the patient needs so that the patient may make an informed decision. The practitioner should impart the information in a sensitive manner, recognising that it might cause distress. The patient must be given time to

consider the information before being required to give the consent unless it is an emergency situation.

2. In many instances the practitioner involved in obtaining informed consent would be a registered medical practitioner. In those circumstances it is the medical practitioner who should impart the information and subsequently seek the signed consent. Normally, in respect of patients in hospital, there are good reasons why the information should be given and the consent sought in the presence of a nurse, midwife or health visitor. Where the procedure or test is to be performed by a nurse, midwife or health visitor the standards described in the preceding paragraph apply to the consent sought.

3. If the nurse, midwife or health visitor does not feel that sufficient information has been given in terms readily understandable to the patient so as to enable him to make a truly informed decision, it is for her to state this opinion and seek to have the situation remedied. The practitioner might decide not to co-operate with a procedure if convinced that the decision to agree to it being performed was not truly informed. Discussion of such matters between the health professionals concerned should not take place in the presence of patients.

   In certain situations and with certain client groups the practitioner's level of responsibility in this respect is greatly increased where she stands in 'loco parentis' for a patient or client.

4. There are occasions on which, although the patient has been given information by the medical practitioner about an intended procedure for which he has given consent, his subsequent statements and questions to a nurse, midwife or health visitor indicate a failure to understand what is to be done, its risks and its ramifications. Where this proves to be the case it is necessary for that practitioner, in the patient's interest, to recall the relevant medical practitioner so that the deficiencies can be remedied without delay.

   The purpose of this approach is to ensure that all professional practitioners involved in the patient's care respect the primacy of that patient's interests, honour their personal professional accountability and avoid the risk of complaint or charges of assault. The practitioner who properly fulfils her responsibilities in this respect should be recognised by medical colleagues as a source of support and information to improve the overall care of the patient.

5. The concept of informed consent and that of truth telling are closely related. If it is to be believed that, on occasions, practitioners withhold information from their patients the damage to public trust and confidence in the profession, on which the introduction to the Code of Professional Conduct places great emphasis, will be enormous.

6. This is yet another area in which judgements have to be made and introduces another facet of the exercise of accountability. If it is accepted that the patient has a right to information about his condition it follows that the professional practitioners involved in his care have a duty to provide such information. Recognition of the patient's condition and the

likely effect of the information might lead the professionals to be selective about 'what' and 'when' but the responsibility is on them to provide information. There may be occasions on which, after consultation with the relatives of a patient by the health professionals involved in that patient's care, some information is temporarily withheld. If, however, something less than the whole truth is told at a particular point in time it should never be because the practitioner is unable to cope with the effects of telling the whole truth. Such controlled release of information (i.e. less than the whole truth) should only ever be in the interests of the patient, and the practitioner should be able to justify the action taken.

7. It is recognised that this is an area in which there is the potential for conflict between professionals involved in the care of the same patient or client. The existence of good, trusting relationships between professionals concerned will promote the development of agreed approaches to truth telling. This subject should be discussed between all the professional practitioners involved so that the rights of patients are not affected adversely. This should minimise the number of occasions on which, after a patient or client has been given incomplete information, a nurse, midwife or health visitor is faced with a request for the whole truth. Accountability can never be exercised by ignoring the rights and interests of the patient or client.

E. Advocacy on behalf of patients and clients

1. The introductory paragraphs of the Code of Professional Conduct, together with several of its clauses, indicate clearly the expectation that the practitioner will accept a role as an advocate on behalf of his or her patients/clients. Opinions vary as to what exactly that means. Some tend to want to identify advocacy as a separate and distinct subject. It is not. It is a component of many professional activities of this and other professions. Some of these professional activities are the subject of other sections of this document.

2. Advocacy is concerned with promoting and safeguarding the wellbeing and interests of patients and clients. It is not concerned with conflict for its own sake. It is important that this fact is recognised, since some practitioners seem to regard advocacy on behalf of patients or clients as an adversarial activity and feel either attracted to it or not able to accept it for that reason. Dictionaries define an advocate as 'one who pleads the cause of another' or 'one who recommends or urges something' and indicates that advocacy is a positive, constructive activity.

3. There are occasions on which the practitioner's advocacy role has to be exercised to 'plead the cause of another' where, in the case of any person incapable of making informed decisions, the parents or relatives withhold consent for treatment which the various practitioners involved believe to be in the best interests of the patient. The parents or relatives, from their knowledge of the patient, will also have an opinion as to what

constitutes his or her best interests. There have been a limited number of cases in which the courts have taken the view that the parents or relatives have not decided in the patient's best interests. Taking the right of decision away from the parents or relatives should only occur in the rarest of cases. The practitioner's advocacy role in situations of this kind requires knowledge of the patient's condition and prognosis, sensitivity to the feelings of the parents or relatives and considerable empathy.

4. To fulfil the Council's expectations set out in the Code is, therefore, to be the advocate for the patient or client in this sense. Each practitioner must determine exactly how this aspect of personal professional accountability is satisfied within her particular sphere of practice. This requires the exercise of judgement as to the 'when' and 'how'. The practitioner must be sure that it is the interests of the patient or client that are being promoted rather than the patient or client being used as a vehicle for the promotion of personal or sectional professional interests. The Code of Professional Conduct envisages the role of patient or client advocate as an integral and essential aspect of good professional practice.

5. Just as the practice of nursing involves the practitioner in assisting the patient with those physical activities which he would do for himself were he able, so too the exercise of professional accountability involves the practitioner in assisting the patient by making such representations on his behalf as he would make himself if he were able.

F. Collaboration and co-operation in care

1. Clause 5 of the Code of Professional Conduct requires that 'Each registered nurse, midwife and health visitor, in the exercise of professional accountability shall work in a collaborative and co-operative manner with other health care professionals and recognise and respect their particular contributions within the health care team'. This clause deliberately emphasises the importance of collaboration and co-operation and, by implication, the importance of the avoidance of dispute and the promotion of good relationships and a spirit of co-operation and mutual respect within the team.

2. It does so because it is clearly impossible for any one profession or agency to possess all the knowledge, skill and resources to be employed in meeting the total health care needs of society. The delivery of full and appropriate care to patients/clients frequently necessitates the participation of professional practitioners from more than one profession, their efforts often being supplemented by other agencies and persons.

   The UKCC recognises the complexity of medical and health care and stresses the need to appreciate the complementary contribution of the professions and others involved.

   The delivery of care is therefore often a multi-profession and multi-agency activity which, in order to be effective, must be based on mutual understanding, trust, respect and co-operation.

3. It is self-evident that collaborative and co-operative working is essential if

patients and clients are to be provided with the care they need and if it is to be of the quality required. It is worthy of note that this concept of teamwork is evident in many situations in which the care of patients and clients is a shared responsibility. Unfortunately there are exceptions. Experience has demonstrated that such co-operation and collaboration is not always easily achieved if: –

(a) individual members of the team have their own specific and separate objectives; or

(b) one member of the team seeks to adopt a dominant role to the exclusion of the opinions, knowledge and skill of its other members.

In such circumstances it is important to stress that the interests of the patient or client must remain paramount.

4. The UKCC and the General Medical Council agree that there is a range of issues which calls for co-operation between the professions at both national and local level and wish to encourage this co-operation.

5. In spite of acceptance of the importance of co-operation and collaboration, differences can sometimes occur within the team regarding appropriate care and treatment. Such conflict can become an influence for good if it results in full discussion between members of the team. It may prove harmful to the care and treatment of patients or clients unless resolved in a manner which recognises the special contribution of each professional group, agency and individual and ensures that the interests and needs of the patient or client remain paramount.

6. Collaboration and co-operation between health care professionals is also necessary in both research and planning related to the provision or improvement of services. This may sometimes give rise to concern where one professional group is requested to pass information (obtained by its members in the course of professional practice) to a member of another professional group to use for a purpose other than that for which it was obtained and recorded. That level of concern will inevitably rise unless it can be seen that the purpose for which the information is required is valid, the information is made available only to persons bound by the same standards of confidentiality and the means of storage and that information is secure.

This should not present a problem where consent can be obtained from the patients or clients to whom the information relates or from relatives who have been provided with the relevant information. In certain fields, such as care of the elderly and persons with mental illness and mental handicap, the information gathering and research geared to the provision of services for these client groups may need to proceed without specific consent. This should only occur where the individuals receiving care are unable to give informed consent and where there is no close contact with relatives. Those who proceed without consent in these particular circumstances must be satisfied that their activities will not affect the current provision of care adversely and that the activity is directed to the provision of appropriate or improved services for future recipients of care.

It is anticipated that disputes will be avoided by relevant inter-professional discussions in advance of submissions of the projects for approval by the appropriate ethical committees. Where a dispute does arise it should be resolved between colleagues and the ethical committee.

Clause 9 of the Code of Professional Conduct and the UKCC's Advisory Paper on 'Confidentiality' provide further sources of reference for nurses, midwives and health visitors in respect of this aspect of practice.

G. *Objection to participation in care and treatment*

1. Clause 7 of the Code of Professional Conduct states:

   'Make known to an appropriate person or authority any conscientious objection which may be relevant to professional practice.'

2. The law does not provide a general opportunity for practitioners to register a conscientious objection to participation in care and treatment. That right applies in respect of termination of pregnancy only (not the care of the patient thereafter) under the terms of Section 4 of the Abortion Act 1967.

3. Some practitioners choose not to participate in certain other forms of treatment on the grounds of conscience. Since the law provides no basic right to such a refusal it is imperative that any practitioner should be careful not to accept employment in a post where it is known that a form of treatment to which she has a conscientious objection is regularly used. In circumstances where a practitioner finds that a form of treatment to which she objects, but which is not usually employed, is to be used she must declare that objection with sufficient time for her managers to make alternative staffing arrangements and must not refuse to participate in emergency treatment.

   Some practitioners may object to participation in certain forms of treatment, such as resuscitative treatment of the elderly, the transfusion of blood, or electro-convulsive therapy. These practitioners must respect clause 7 of the Code and make their position clear to their professional colleagues and managers, and recognise that this may have implications for their contract of employment.

4. Objection to participation in treatment does not only occur as a product of conscience. It is the Council's stated position that, on each and every occasion a prescribed medication is being administered, the practitioner should ensure that, in her view, the patient is not presenting symptoms that contra-indicate its administration. The practitioner who is concerned about the administration of a particular drug in these circumstances might reasonably ask the prescribing doctor to attend the patient and, if the prescriber still requires it to be given, to request her to administer the medication if not fully reassured. The practitioner involved in such an incident should make a detailed record of the reasons why she felt concern and, if so, why she declined to administer prescribed medication.

5. The principle that applies in the previous paragraph can also be applied

in appropriate circumstances to substances that are prescribed for topical use including wound dressings. Where the practitioner attending the patient believes (from knowledge, published research evidence or from previous experience) that the prescribed substance may be harmful, or even more so where it is evident that it is actively harmful, she should make a record of the condition of the wound or site (where appropriate including a photographic record) and ask the prescribing medical practitioner to attend.

If the prescription stands after medical examination the practitioner, having chosen either to respond to the prescription or not, should make a detailed record of the reasons for her expressed concern and subsequent actions.

It is believed that the spirit of co-operation and mutual respect referred to in paragraph F1. of this document should make such situations exceptional.

6. Objections to participation in treatment are not always associated with the nature or form of treatment or its appropriateness in a particular set of circumstances. Some practitioners indicate their wish or active intention to refuse to participate in the delivery of care to patients with certain conditions. Such refusal may be associated particularly with patients suffering from Hepatitis B Infection and those with Acquired Immune Deficiency Syndrome, AIDS Related Complex or who are HIV seropositive but asymptomatic.

Those who seek the UKCC's support for such actual or intended refusal are informed that the Code of Professional Conduct does not provide a formula for being selective about the categories of patient or client for whom the practitioner will care. To seek to be so selective is to demonstrate unacceptable conduct. The UKCC expects its practitioners to adopt a non-judgemental approach in the exercise of their caring role.

H. Summary of the principles against which to exercise accountability

1. The interests of the patient or client are paramount.
2. Professional accountability must be exercised in such a manner as to ensure that the primacy of the interests of patients or clients is respected and must not be overridden by those of the professions or their practitioners.
3. The exercise of accountability requires the practitioner to seek to achieve and maintain high standards.
4. Advocacy on behalf of patients or clients is an essential feature of the exercise of accountability by a professional practitioner.
5. The role of other persons in the delivery of health care to patients or clients must be recognised and respected, provided that the first principle above is honoured.

6. Public trust and confidence in the profession is dependent on its practitioners being seen to exercise their accountability responsibly.
7. Each registered nurse, midwife or health visitor must be able to justify any action or decision not to act taken in the course of her professional practice.

Index